Blurbs

This is a book about food, home, belonging, travel, friendship—all the things that make us who we are. But above all it's a book about family, faith, and love and the widest, most generous and all-embracing definitions of all of them. It also tells a story of the Indian diaspora, how a small family grew and spread, weaving itself into other countries and cultures near and far, making contributions wherever it went, but always remembering where it came from and what that teaches us. As a member of the vast cousinage it lovingly describes, it filled me with a deep sense of pride. But it's also a funny, moving, and deeply inspiring book.

Philip Pothen
Kent University Educator, author, and cousin, UK

The Bear Wore a Swimsuit is a charming memoir narrated by Dr Susie Baboo Samuel that chronicles the fascinating story of her family and her early life in colonial Singapore. Trained at the prestigious Christian Medical College and Hospital Vellore, India, and at St John's Hospital, London, Susie worked for the Leprosy Mission International in Bhutan and Nepal and shares her experiences of treating one of the world's oldest diseases, which has traumatised humankind. Susie's autobiography is a must-read for lovers of family dramas, sagas, and love stories!

Usha Jesudasan
Author, India

A striking account, with a refreshing light touch, from one who shared the family life shaped by her father's conviction that the Church, the bride of Christ with all her warts and pimples, still has first priority in a pastor's life. The recorded humanness of the divine call will warm & encourage your heart.

Rt Rev Rennis Ponniah
A Christ Church kid and her pride and joy, is the retired 9th Bishop of Singapore & Hon Director of Global South Fellowship of Anglican Churches, Singapore

I am delighted to know that this book has finally arrived. I have known the author, Dr Susie Samuel for almost six decades, starting with medical college. Even among a class of sixty students, which includes several distinguished public speakers and a few published authors, Susie has a special place.

During our days in the hostel, she would share stories of her childhood in Singapore, her many accomplished and eccentric relatives, and more. Then, as we followed her through postgraduate studies in specialties as diverse as obstetrics, gynaecology, and dermatology and her work in Nepal, Bhutan, UK, and back in India, we continued to be enthralled by her stories.

She has forayed into the world of fashion design, cooking, baking, gardening, and philanthropy. And she has continued to collect and share her experiences, to a chorus of '*Susie, must write a book*'. And finally, the book is here.

Congratulations, Susie, and may your fan following increase.

Dr Joyce Ponnaiya
Med School Classmate, CMC, Vellore, Batch of 1964
Former Principal & Director, Christian Medical College Vellore, India

The Bear Wore a Swimsuit

The Bear Wore a Swimsuit

Dr Susie Baboo Samuel

Vitasta

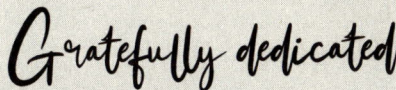
Gratefully dedicated

To all our teachers at St Margaret's School
Especially our English teachers
Miss Isabel Lau,
Mrs Phyllis Chin,
& Mrs Sushila Appadurai Cherian
And
Mrs Martha Holloway, our beloved Principal
who in her infinite wisdom decided on the white
coat for me.

Published by
Vitasta Publishing Pvt Ltd
2/15, Ansari Road, Daryaganj
New Delhi - 110 002
info@vitastapublishing.com

ISBN: 978-81-963329-8-3

© Dr Susie Baboo Samuel

First Edition 2023

MRP ₹495

All Rights Reserved.

No part of this publication may be reproduced, stored in a retrieval system, or transmitted in any form, or by any means – electronic, mechanical, photocopying, recording or otherwise – without the prior permission of the publisher.

The author pledges the royalties from the sale of the book to The Banyan. https://thebanyan.org
The Banyan is a non-governmental organisation based in Chennai that offers comprehensive mental health and social care services to mentally ill and homeless women in the city.

Cover Design by Vincent M Raja
Photo credit by Konica Colour Lab
Typeset by Somesh Kumar MISHRA
Printed at Chaman Enterprises, New Delhi

Contents

Foreword xi
Introduction xiii
Prologue xv
A story that almost never happened xvii

Part 1 1-28
    ....My Annammal Paatti 1
Part 2 29-80
    The war years 30
Part 3 81-99
    Retired and Relocated 82
Part 4 100-162
    St Margaret's School 101
Part 5 163-192
    For better, for worse 164
Part 6 193-262
    The sadness in their eyes 194

Thank you.. 263
Epilogue 287

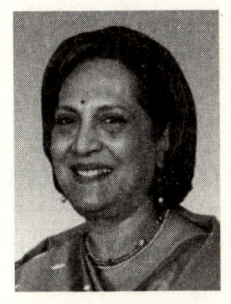

Foreword

The title of Dr Susie Samuel's memoir, *The Bear wore a Swimsuit*, prepares the reader for a humour-infused journey through her life and experiences as a doctor and much more. There are elements of everything that make for a thoroughly enjoyable read.

There is history, mystery, and suspense with a happy ending to the love story of her parents. There are lively accounts of her own childhood in Singapore and then travels across the globe with her wonderful husband, Sam and children, Rekha and Anish. And, there are many, both serious and funny, stories of a large community of relatives, friends, pets, and patients whom she gathered around her, including my parents.

Stitching all the strands of the narration of a remarkable life together is a strong skein of empathy and a style of writing which captivates with its simple and direct style.

—**Deepa Wadhwa**

Deepa Gopalan Wadhwa, IFS, is a career diplomat who retired after serving as an Ambassador of India to Japan, Qatar, and Sweden with significant assignments in China, The Netherlands, India's Permanent Mission to the UN at Geneva, the International Labour Organization (ILO), and the Ministry of External Affairs. Ms Wadhwa is currently the Chairperson of the India-Japan Friendship Forum and works with think tanks related to foreign policies.

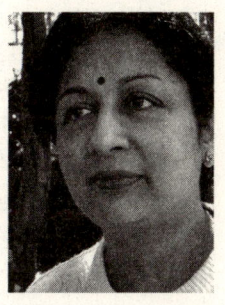

Introduction

This book very nearly did not reach the printer because exactly like Life, it kept being pummelled either by the writer or by the publisher.

The elegant team that worked on it a *yuga* ago gave up worrying about it the way a midwife goes home after the baby is in the arms of its mother, but this baby refused to stay in its swaddling clothes and kept trying to return to the womb for this or that beautification.

This endlessly entertaining book is valuable for two reasons. One, it is an honest account and assessment of a remarkable life lived with humour and compassion. Two, Susie Samuel should have been a full-time writer. Somehow the stars over her cradle aligned in such a fashion that she ended up studying medicine. It is a mirror to the personality who gives away her professional gifts gratis and throws a protective net over everyone who comes her way. Before there were books, there were stories. At first the stories were not written down. Sometimes they were sung. Before they could speak, children listened to their parents singing to them or telling stories about an egg that fell off a wall or a girl who fell down a rabbit hole. The books and the stories we begin to live with make us who we are. Everything we read changes us in some way, hence the ancient warning, not to read or view indiscriminately.

I would advise everyone to be indiscriminate about reading Susie's life writing because they can only be changed for the better for the adventure that awaits them.

—**Mini Krishnan**

Mini Krishnan, a visionary in the publishing world, is the face of translations in India. In her four-decade-long illustrious career in publishing with Macmillan and Oxford University Press, Mini Krishnan has edited and brought to life 135 translations-fiction, non-fiction, poetry, and short stories-from 14 languages, been a member of several award and advisory panels, and worked on educational texts prescribed at school and university levels. She is currently an adviser to the Tamil Nadu Government, coordinating translation.

Prologue

A story that almost never happened. My Dad was presumed dead during the Japanese occupation of Singapore during WW-II. When he returned unannounced to India many weary and incommunicado years later, no one recognised him. Not even my Mum, who had assumed that she was a war widow. Only his faithful K9, a German Shepherd named Sundar, did.

I... A story that almost never happened

My Mum was nearly forty-five when the Second World War, WW-II, separated her from my Dad and left them stranded on either side of the Indian Ocean: My Mum in Madras and my Dad in Singapore. When my Dad left my Mum in the Madras Medical College to finish her medical studies and sailed to Singapore to assume charge of the Tamil congregation Christ Church, he never dreamt that it would be many turbulent years before they found each other again. They had found love late, only to lose it.

After she graduated, my Mum booked her passage on a ship plying between Madras and Singapore. Her excitement at the thought of joining my Dad after all the years apart was cut short by the ominous clouds of WW-II. On 15th February 1942, Japanese troops defeated the combined troops of the British, the Australians, the Indians, and the Malays to conquer the island of Singapore and renamed it *Syonan* for the Japanese occupation from 1942-45. A few days later, the ship slated to carry my Mum to Singapore was hit by Japanese airstrikes, disrupting travel between Singapore and Madras. The damaged vessel sank to the bottom of the coast of Singapore together with my Mum's plans of joining my Dad. Though there was absolutely no communication between them, my Mum never forgot the gentle priest who had answered a call to service overseas. For many months, my Mum had absolutely no idea if my Dad was dead or alive, imprisoned or free. Her parents had died by then, and she would have been utterly alone if her siblings had not formed a protective band around her, sharing their lives and their families with her.

They watched helplessly as the silence of every passing day helped convince my Mum that she had been widowed. They knew how much she loved her coloured silks, puff-sleeve blouses, matching accessories, and the scented jasmine flowers she wore in her hair. They cried silent tears when she took to wearing white as Christian widows were wont to do and stopped wearing flowers in her hair. My Mum stepped into several years of presumed widowhood vacillating between numbing fear and exhilarating hope in what must have been the saddest and toughest trough of her life; when she had to hide her sorrow from her family who looked to her for courage and comfort. She found it hard to accept her loss without any confirmation, even as she continued to hope against hope.

My Mum joined the Tamil Nadu government health services after she passed her MBBS from Madras Medical College and was posted to Cuddalore, a tiny fishing village on the southern coast of India, where she threw herself into her work as a Medical Officer at the government hospital. She may have spent the better part of the night crying softly into her pillow in the privacy of her bedroom, but when the sun rose, she put on a brave face for the world and her family. Every morning, my Mum would leave for work with her stethoscope in her coat pocket and a bottle of drinking water and two ripe bananas for her mid-morning coffee break in a wicker basket.

She would cover the short walk between her staff quarters and the outpatient veranda of the hospital with Sundar, my Dad's Alsatian, shuffling alongside as her bodyguard. Having him close to her was a great source of comfort as it gave her a glimmer of hope that my Dad would return someday. Sundar never left my Mum's side. It was almost as if my Dad had left him to watch over her.

My Dad loved dogs, and Sundar was a mere puppy when he sailed to Singapore. When my Mum was staying in the hostel in Madras, unable to keep pets, she had left Sundar with her siblings, the *Cadavanaltharayil* family in Kodukulanji, a hamlet up in the hills of central Travancore, which later became part of Kerala. When she finished her course and found that her plans of sailing to Singapore had sunk, she took Sundar with her to Cuddalore. Sundar, meanwhile, had grown old and weary waiting for his master's return. While she worked, he would sleep at her feet under her chair with his wet nose pressed against her foot, not stirring except for the occasional reassuring nuzzle to let her know that he was there with her, moving only when she got up to leave.

One afternoon, when my Mum was working at the clinic, a man appeared at the hospital to see her. It was a hot and dusty day in the busy outpatient clinic, and there was a long line of patients waiting to be seen. No one was in a good mood nor were they pleased with the patient, who did not seem to be from these parts, when he jumped the queue. Ignoring their angry protests, he pushed his way to the front of the line as if his life depended on it. He did not say a word. Nor did he tell the nurse his name when asked. He just pushed past her and made a beeline for the doctor's table and stood staring long and hard at her, his eyes bright with unshed tears. He seemed quite emotional as he stumbled and would have fallen if he had not placed both his hands on her table for support. A long salt-and-pepper beard hung from his gaunt face, and he seemed extremely weary as if he had reached the end of a long and exhausting journey.

Preoccupied with another patient, my Mum looked up impatiently at the man before her who had pushed his way through the restive crowd in the outpatient hall. Something about him was vaguely familiar. She thought she had seen him somewhere before. Suddenly, Sundar, who was fast asleep under her chair, came alive. Barking furiously, he shot out from under her chair and flung himself at the stranger who had dropped down onto his knees on the floor beside her chair. For a moment, my Mum wondered if Sundar was attacking the stranger. Confused and slightly alarmed, she looked down at the man and dog greet each other with unbridled joy. My Mum could not fathom this atypical behaviour. *What on earth is wrong with Sundar?* she wondered. *Why is he jumping up and down like a lunatic?* Arthritic and near blind, Sundar was usually completely indifferent to strangers. He related only to my Mum, not even to the siblings and their families. She looked up at the man curiously, still unable to place him. It was only when he smiled that she recognised him in a flash. It was my Dad.

My Dad had survived the horrors of the war and had come home to my Mum - truly a fairy tale ending to their cruel separation.

A miracle

When my Dad sailed back to Singapore, my Mum could not accompany him as they found that they were expecting a baby. Singapore was slowly limping back to normalcy after the war-ravaged years, and the health services were in disarray.

Therefore, they decided that the best option was for my Mum to stay back in India for the birth of their child. They were as delighted as they were fearful, stunned by this miracle after all they had gone through. I was born on 16th November 1946 when my Mum was around forty-six, narrowly missing every possible congenital deformity and complication listed in the chapter on the elderly primigravida and high-risk pregnancies.

My Mum went back to CMC, the Christian Medical College Vellore, her alma mater where she had started her medical studies, for her delivery as she anticipated complications that might need skilled obstetric/neonatal care and intervention. Though it was a premature delivery, there were mercifully no complications.

When my Mum returned to Cuddalore, she was flooded with visitors. They were delighted that the Lady Doctor, who had believed that she was a war widow for so many years, was now a mother with an infant in her arms. The family was overjoyed that my Mum had been blessed with a baby. My Dad's Mum, *Annammal Paatti*, was over the moon when she heard the news as she had given up all hope of ever becoming a grandmother.

Among Malayalees, the first child is usually named after the father's parents, depending on the gender of the baby, while the second child is named after the mother's parents. Since I was a flash-in-the-pan and the chances of a replay seemed highly unlikely, I was christened Anne Elizabeth after both my grandmothers and answered to Susie all my life. A few weeks after my baptism in Cuddalore, the three of us—my Mum, my Aunt Esther (sibling no. 17), and I—sailed to Singapore where my Dad was waiting at the harbour to receive us, beaming from ear to ear.

Susie the baby, carried off that boat, was the product of her genetic influences. Susie the adult who is telling you her story is, on the other hand, the result of all the places she lived in, the people she interacted with, the education she was blessed to receive, the circumstances she survived, and the lessons she learned.

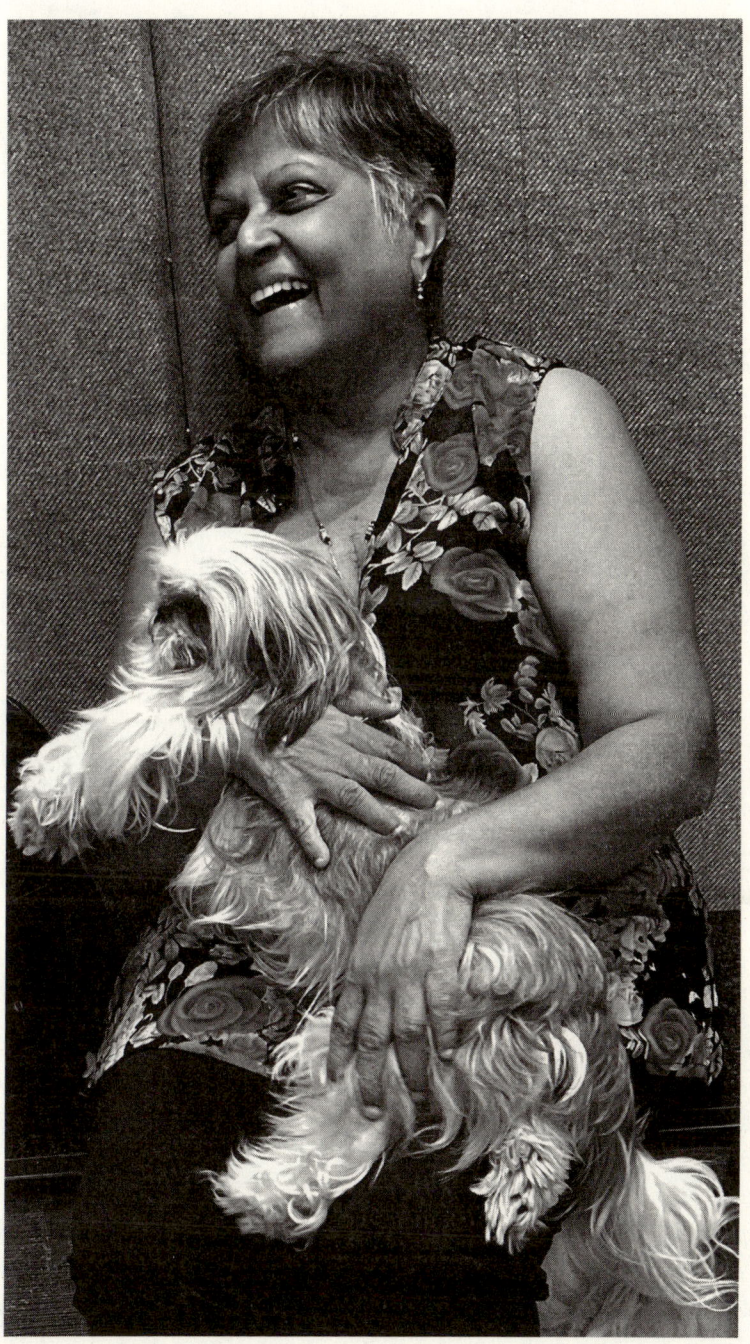

PART 1

Grandparents | The Cadavanaltharayils | Parents

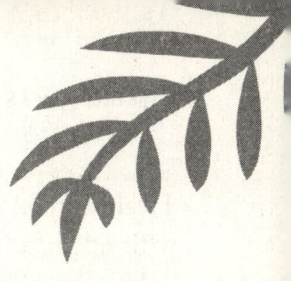

.....My Annammal Paatti

My Dad's mother, my *Annammal Paatti*, was widowed young with two children—my Dad and his sister, Alice—siblings she raised as a single Mum in the tiny village of Senthiambalam near Tuticorin in South India. I do not know much about my Dad's father, my *Samuel Thatha*, who passed away as a young man early in the marriage when my Dad was just a toddler.

One grandmother like my *Annammal Paatti* is enough for a million grandchildren. A powerhouse of love, she gave it all to me, her only grandchild, to cherish and stow away for this lifetime and the next. Mention her name and I see a tall, long-boned, silver-haired lady with a slight stoop, a toothless smile, and pure, undiluted love shining brightly from her sightless eyes. Mention her name and a cascade of warm and tender memories come tumbling out. Mention her name and I feel a happy, fuzzy glow inside me: a feel-good feeling that feels really good!

While chopping firewood as a young mother, a splinter flew into my *Annammal Paatti*'s right eye, a horrendous accident that led to the painful loss of vision on the right side.

Healthcare in Senthiambalam was abysmal, and within weeks, a florid infection set in to herald sympathetic ophthalmitis, robbing my *Annammal Paatti* of sight in both eyes leaving her struggling as a young widow and a single Mum. A darkened world and two small children hanging on to her helpless hands on either side did not keep her down for too long. It only strengthened her faith in *Yesu Christu,* the Risen Saviour, who never left her side.

Yesu Christu was not just another name in her old Tamil Bible that her neighbours took turns to read out to her. He did not pop up once in a while or when called upon on Sundays and at prayer meetings. He was a living presence in her life, a daily companion who never left her side. She trusted Him implicitly. She leaned on Him totally. She consulted Him. She complained to Him. She joked with Him. She thanked Him, and she worshipped Him. He lived in her heart, and she took Him everywhere she went. Her faith in her living saviour was simple, childlike, and absolute. Her faith in *Yesu Christu* kept her alive and well for ninety-nine years. I was in medical college when she left me, taking a part of me with her forever.

My dear, sweet *Annammal Paatti*.

After her children left home, my *Annammal Paatti* lived a fairly independent life, under the watchful eyes of the loving village. Her home, the Prayer House—a white building on the mud road leading to the quaint St Mark's Church in Senthiambalam—was never locked and was always left open for the villagers. People dropped in for prayers, be it for a sick child, for a journey, or just for a blessing. Just about anything really. She knew more secrets than anyone else in the village as they all trusted her. Perhaps her blindness gave them some degree of immunity during their confessions. Over the years, she acquired the name *Jebam Panre Paatti*, the *Grandmother*

Who Prays, a name she is remembered by in the village even today.

She never saw my Dad or his sister as adults. She had no idea what her daughter-in-law or her only grandchild looked like. As a child, on our annual holidays, I remember lying in her lap while she traced every contour of my face.

Every evening, she would string fragrant jasmine flowers, gathered from her garden, for my hair. Putting me on her lap with my back to her, she would comb my hair and braid it, intertwining the string of jasmine flowers into my plaits. It was a ritual with her, while I sat fidgeting, waiting impatiently to run out and play with the other kids.

She never ever called me by my name, only various terms of endearment in *Tamizh*. One that she used often was *Yennai Petra Thaiye*. When I asked her what it meant, she told me that it meant *Oh mother who gave me life* in *Tamizh*. I rather liked that. I did not understand the depth or enormity of the endearment; it just made me feel cherished. Every time she said it, I grew a few inches taller. Decades later, I can still remember quite distinctly the tangible love in her voice whenever she spoke to me. No one has loved me as much or as unconditionally as my *Annammal Paatti* did. *No one*.

Whenever we visited her, my *Annammal Paatti* would cure goat meat for us to take back to Singapore. Fat-free pieces of meat cubed with amazing precision, marinated in turmeric and rock salt, would be strung on a twine and dried like clothes on a wash line, outside during the day and inside during the night. After a few days in the blazing sun closely guarded by someone with a stick to shoo off pesky crows, the dried cubes of meat would be tied across the storeroom behind the kitchen and left to dry out completely. Later, the dried meat, the famous *attu kari uppukandam*, would be stripped off the twine and packed into roomy airtight biscuit tins for us to take home to Singapore. This happened every visit and she never paid attention when my Dad protested that we had the best Australian lamb in Singapore.

Humouring him, she would make suitable noises. *Hmmmm... Appidiya? Is that so? Uh Huh. Really?* never looking up from what she was doing. The best of Australian lamb did not impress my *Annammal Paatti*. I doubt if she even knew of Australia or where it was on the map. We always took the cured meat back with us, respecting the love that went into the act.

My Velliammachy

My Mum's mother, my *Velliammachy*, passed away before I was born. I only have a treasure trove of stories that we, her fifty-eight grandchildren, were raised on. When my *Velliammachy*, Aleyamma Mathan, got married, she was barely fifteen. Her father, Rev. MP Mathan from the *Tholaserry Molomootil* family in Thiruvalla, was a Church Missionary Society pastor. Growing up in the parsonage with her parents and siblings, *Velliammachy* blossomed into a lively tomboy her mother despaired over. There was not a tree around the house she had not climbed alongside her brothers with her skirt tucked securely between her legs, freeing her to effortlessly scale up or down the trunks, often reaching heights they could not.

She wielded a slingshot better than her brothers did and brought down fruits faster than they could. She could whistle louder than her brothers and fish better than they could. Anything her brothers did, she could do better. Not in the slightest bit domesticated, she was happiest playing or working outside. She did not enjoy slaving over the kitchen stove, nor did the needle and thread enthral her. She would never have learned cooking had she not been tied up in the kitchen on a regular basis.

Wheat-complexioned, her elfin face capped by a widow's peak, and her thick, jet-black braid swinging defiantly about her, she seemed to be in a hurry all the time, running instead of walking sedately as her mother would have wanted. Eyes dancing with mischief, she smiled impishly at the world as she skated in and out of trouble. Though her spirited ways and impudence endeared her to the family and neighbours, her mother, my great-grandmother, worried about how she would ever fit into her husband's home after marriage.

Having noticed the young Aleyamma in church one day, a relative met her father with a marriage proposal. *Mathan Achen* conferred with his wife, and a date was set for a viewing session, *the pennu kaannaan* visit, when the matchmaker would bring the boy and his family—the boy's people—home to see their daughter.

Arranged marriages

Marriages might well be made in heaven, but match-making is definitely done on earth. Marriages were usually arranged either by a professional or by a member of the family with a fertile imagination. Normally, prospective brides were checked by a motley crew of relatives, both close and distant, and others who tagged along for the ride.

As soon as the entourage was spotted in the village, the girl's family would be alerted that the boy's people were on their way. The visitors would be welcomed and pleasantries exchanged after which the girl would be called in to serve tea and nibbles that the family claimed were made by her. If you ate with gusto, it meant that you liked the girl. If there were reservations, the visitors would exercise polite restraint when the food came around.

One of my cousins got into serious trouble because of the lack of restraint he showed over the food that he was served on his *pennu kannaan* visits. To be fair, he had only just come home after working for years in a cold Scandinavian country languishing on a bland continental diet. Starved of all his favourite dishes, he longed for the curries cooked in the wood-fired, earthenware pots in his mother's kitchen. Seeing the food on the viewing rounds, he thought he had died and gone to heaven. Without looking up from his plate, he ate up everything he was offered and anything else he clapped eyes on, sending wrong signals of approval to the girl's family. Later, out of earshot, when he was asked if he liked the girl, he mumbled, *What girl? Where girl? I only saw the food.* Eventually, he was muzzled and kept on a short leash until his yearning palate calmed down sufficiently to make the right choice.

During the *pennu kaannaan* visit, the nervous girl under inspection would be pushed into the room with the tea tray. A mental note would be made of her gait and stance to see if she had a limp or deformity. Her weight would be recorded on an invisible scale. Thin was out. Fat, considered healthy, was in. She would be asked to read out verses from the Bible, to rule out a stammer. Musical achievements were a bonus and looks though important, were secondary. She had to be healthy and strong to run the house and bear children. If you slipped through the nets and fell in love, that was different. But if you were seeking an alliance in the arranged marriage market, you went shopping; you inspected the goods and chose the best you could. The lives of two young people depended on the choices made for them at the viewing. After the covert but rigorous inspection, the visitors would leave, promising to call later with an answer. There was however no guarantee that the same girl seen at home during the viewing would walk up the steps to the church. Old maids, spinster sisters of the bride, shrouded heavily in bridal saris, have been known to step off the shelf to appear at the altar, at a point of no return.

Sometimes, the boy and girl never met at all before the wedding. They met for the first time at the altar, in an act of faith, during the wedding ceremony. Perfect strangers vowed to stay together forever till death did them part. Growing up, you were not allowed to speak to strangers of the opposite sex. But it was perfectly okay to marry one and jump into bed with them, provided the family found them for you.

Many of these marriages lasted several long and happy years, ending only with the death of a partner. Expectations in arranged marriages are akin to the psychological response in the *Stockholm syndrome,* where hostages empathise with their captors and develop positive feelings towards them, even defending them fiercely when love peeped in to stay. The elders in the family shortlisted and fine-tuned the process of finding a suitable match. The boy and girl simply did as they were told. They dressed up when it was time, walked down to the local church in their new clothes, and got married.

My Velliappachan

The young man shortlisted to view Aleyamma was CP John, one of the sons of *Potha Upadeshi*, a catechist from the *Cheruvadekilil* family. Though he had graduated with flying colours from the CMS College in Kottayam, he settled down to teach at the Kodukulanji High School because his family could not afford to educate him any further. A committed Christian, he spent most of his spare time preaching the gospel to the labourers, the untouchables in the caste tier, who worked in the rice fields for the landed gentry. Well respected amongst his peers, he was considered a suitable match for *Mathan Achen's* daughter, Aleyamma.

My *Velliammachy* was irritated that her morning capers

were interrupted by the visit of the boy's people. Plucked off the branches of the mango tree, she was sent to wash up and get ready. Protesting bitterly all the way, she entered the viewing room armed with a tea tray and nibbles, scowling and muttering under her breath. Tripping over slippers she rarely wore, she looked up and saw a handsome man with kind eyes, at least ten years older than her, watching her with an amused expression. Young CP John knew that life would never be the same again. He knew that he would never have a dull moment if he married Aleyamma, the vivacious girl he had come to see. The rest is history. As newlyweds, they moved into *Cadavanaltharayil* - a house near a banyan tree, by the canal in Kodukulanji. In a dramatic switch, my *Velliammachy* went from a tomboy climbing trees to a child bride and wife. Living out an obstetric miracle spanning twenty-eight reproductive years, she delivered nineteen children, including a set of twins, at home in her own bed. The village joked about the prolific *Cadavanaltharayils*, who seemed to be everywhere. Over the years, death, disease, and disaster rounded off the survivors to an even dozen who survived beyond the age of fifty.

Veetuperu

You might be wondering how my grandfather CP John, *Cadavanaltharayil* Pothen John, had an unpronounceable name with seventeen letters and no hyphens strung together. He was christened Pothen John - Pothen being the Malayalam equivalent of Paul. That was his name. *Cadavanaltharayil* was his house name, his *veetuperu*, a surname that placed him securely in a clan in Kerala. Even when woken up from deep sleep, the elders in the family could swing effortlessly up and down the branches of the family tree without missing a step to claim kinship and inheritance. The house name was a verbal map of their home. In an era when there were no street names, no house numbers, or pin codes, it identified the location of their home accurately with reference to a fixed, immovable point nearby like a church, a school, a water body, a hillock, or even a tree. If there was mail to be delivered, the *veetuperu* ensured that the letter reached the family. *Cadavanaltharayil* translated into *the house under the banyan tree near a canal*. The girls in the family shed their *veetuperu* to acquire their husband's *veetuperu* when they got married and moved to their new home. In a split second, a Susie could go from a *Susie-Under-the-Mango-Tree* to a *Susie-Under-the-Jackfruit-Tree!*

The boys proudly passed it on to their children as a legacy. Even when they crossed oceans to migrate overseas, they carried the prefix *Cadavanaltharayil* with their name. They shortened it to the letter *C* if there was no space on a dotted line, but they never ever discarded their *veetuperu*. They wore it with pride when alive, and they wore it with pride when it was engraved on their tombstones when they were laid to rest.

My Mum

My Mum, Saramma, the fifth child of her parents, was the eldest of the twelve siblings who crossed fifty birthdays. Her siblings called her *Pengal*, a term usually used by brothers for an elder sister. With four younger brothers in quick succession, the name stuck even when her younger sisters arrived much later. Over the years, she grew to be more than a *Pengal* as she assumed all the duties of a parent. Waking or sleeping, she had only one agenda: the welfare of her siblings and their families. A chronic ear infection left her hearing-challenged as a child. Though her deafness worsened with age and became a part of her life and ours, it never dwarfed her authority. No one dared to defy her, at least not to her face.

Her whole life was a mural of devotion intent on improving the lot of her siblings and their families. They were not expected to return the money spent on their education, but there was an unwritten rule that they would, when prompted, turn around and help the next sibling waiting in the wings. Their family motto could well have read: *Each one help one*. My Mum's muffled world was divided into two hemispheres. One had her siblings behind her protective back and the other, facing her, had the rest of the world – a world she would have taken on at any cost to protect her siblings.

There were some long-standing feuds between the siblings, with undercurrents of doubt and discontent, when they became adults with families of their own. Most of these tiffs that rumbled at family gatherings were connected through serial pages of bookkeeping and accounts. However, there was one golden rule that they never broke. They could fight and bite and scratch amongst themselves, but the world could not touch *any* one of them. If the enemy was from the outside, all twelve siblings would line up, arm in arm, shoulder to shoulder, and take on the outsider. Blood definitely ran thicker than water among the siblings.

Growing up, my Mum was far too preoccupied with her siblings to think of her own life. She completed her LMP, the Licentiate Medical Practitioner's course from CMC Vellore, the Christian Medical College, class of 1925, as one of the first few privileged batches to be taught by Dr Ida Scudder, the visionary who founded the college in 1920. After she graduated and started working as a doctor, she received a string of marriage proposals that eventually petered out when the boy's people realised that she would never leave her siblings. Anyone who married her would automatically inherit her siblings and their families as dowry. She refused to get married as most boys and their families did not want her to continue supporting her family after marriage. Once married, she and her income as a doctor would rightfully belong to her husband and his people. To my Mum this was inconceivable as she would have stopped breathing if she had to turn her back on her siblings!

My Dad

The man who married her would have to allow her to look after her siblings long after the first flush of romance ended. One man loved her enough to share her with her siblings: my Dad, Paramanantham Israel Samuel Baboo, a name my children thought was perfect for anagrams. His mother, my *Annammal Paatti* lived in Senthiambalem and her livelihood came from a piece of land, a garden she referred to as *The Thottam*, a scant half-acre that she owned a short distance from her home. The income from *The Thottam* was all that she had to bring up her two children, my Dad and his sister, and it was a struggle from the word go as the land was dry and arid, barely allowing plantains and groundnuts to grow.

As my Dad did extremely well at school, my *Annammal Paatti* was determined that her son should be allowed to study for as long as he could as she believed that he would do extremely well if given the chance. The one beacon that lit her sightless world was her ambition to see my Dad reach his full potential.

The gender slant was undeniable in the southern states. Boys were more important than girls in all things big and small. Unfortunately, this meant that my Dad and his education became a priority, while my Aunt Alice—my *athai*—remained a mere girl child to be married off when she came of age. I doubt if my aunt was pleased with this preferential treatment. I am sure she felt she could have done just as well as, or better than my Dad, had she been given the same opportunities. As a teenager, she was packed off to grow up with the Millers, my *Annammal Paatti's* cousins in Pune. After she completed her schooling, she trained with a pharmacist and eventually set up a medical shop in Pune. Financially independent, she remained single, running two auto services on the road as a successful entrepreneur.

My Dad was taken by one of his uncles to study in Ambur. He was expected to work in his uncle's fields before and after school in return for his board and lodge. It was an extremely hard life, physically and emotionally. Life as a poor relative at the receiving end is never easy. It is humiliating to be dependent on hand-me-downs and largesse no matter how kind they are meant to be. The only thing no one could ever take away from him was his dignity. Determined to rise above his circumstances, he set about excelling in his studies.

In his twenties, he walked barefoot over muddy rural roads in India, dressed in threadbare clothes. In his sixties, he drove a Mercedes Benz in Singapore. He may have come from humble beginnings, but he rose with God's blessings and sheer hard work to become a self-made man, a scholar, and the most wonderful human being I have ever known. I say this with enormous pride, humbled that he was my Dad.

My Dad never ever forgot his modest beginnings; and he never forgot the taste of hunger. There was one cardinal rule that could never be broken in the parsonage. *No grumbling or crying at the table.* If I fussed at the table, I would be reminded very curtly, that there were millions starving around the world. Years later, when my own kids fussed at the table, I pulled out the *Millions are starving around the world* line from my childhood. Unfortunately, they grew up with more democracy than I did, and I drew a blank when they suggested that I send the bitter gourd and all the other veggies they hated to the starving millions. My cheeky monkeys even offered to help me pack them for despatch!

As the school topper, my Dad was awarded a scholarship to do his BA in the American College in Madurai. Securing a second scholarship after his BA, he went on to study theology at Bishop's College in Calcutta for his BD degree. After my Dad passed away, his friend and colleague Rev. VM Thomas helped me sort out my Dad's library. All the books he had collected with great pride over the years were sent to various theological seminaries, together with his cassocks and vestments to be used by young priests in training, instead of them lying around gathering dust on a shelf. Uncle Thomas showed me a book my Dad had been awarded for the Alexander Prize in Greek at Bishops College on 17th December 1932. I had known my Dad for nearly 40 years but I had absolutely no idea that he had studied Greek or won a prize for it. My Dad had no airs or graces as he moved on in life. He had the kindest and the most disarming smile I have ever seen on a human face. When he smiled, his eyes crinkled and the imposing figure that he cut in his white cassock transformed into everyone's familiar *Baboo Achen,* the *Pathriyar* who broke all records to serve as the vicar of Christ Church in Singapore for thirty-one years.

Sunday lunches at Ettiyapuram

As a young priest, my Dad was posted to several villages in Tamil Nadu. When he was posted to Ettiyapuram, he met a shy Malayalee lady doctor, Saramma John, the resident doctor at the government clinic. My Dad used to cycle around the villages visiting the various parishes under his care. Every Sunday, he would reach the Ettiyapuram Tamil Church mid-morning to conduct their service, which usually finished around noon. The elders in the church felt it was cruel to let him pedal off to the next village in the scorching sun without lunch, so they decided that he should have lunch in one of the homes. Looking around, they agreed that *Doctor Amma's* home was the most suitable, and they requested my Mum to kindly serve him lunch on Sundays.

Though my Mum was single, her home was considered safe for the young priest as *Doctor Amma's* home was always bustling with people. Apparently her large family seemed to be coming and going, visiting or staying with her the year round. If anyone in the family was sick, they came and stayed with her for their treatment. If there was a death in the family, they met at her home to grieve. Newlyweds shared their honeymoon with her, while her home was the vacation destination for the kids in schools and colleges. Being the only doctor in the family, all her sisters and sisters-in-law came to her for their confinement and delivery. She was apparently always well chaperoned as there were at least half a dozen people staying with her at any point in time.

My Mum agreed to look after the visiting priest as it would have been no extra trouble to set another plate at her table, which was, in any case, always full. Little did she know then that the extra plate she set at a Sunday lunch in Ettiyapuram would end up being a permanent fixture at the head of her dining table. She called him *Iyah,* the *Tamizh* term of respect used to address a priest, when she first met him in Ettiyapuram, and she called him *Iyah* until the day she died. Even when she scolded him later on in life, she still called him *Iyah*. *This Iyah is hopeless!* she would exclaim, throwing up her hands in exasperation, hopeless being a favourite word in her vocabulary.

My Mum's family was a warm-hearted bunch that welcomed visitors. They were used to shuffling to accommodate and stretching to share. Excellent cooks, the girls would whip up an impressive spread for the visiting priest on Sundays. As time passed he found himself looking forward to his visits to Ettiyapuram. He was not sure what it was that he enjoyed more: the appreciative congregation, the unfamiliar warmth and hospitality at *Doctor Amma's* house, or the delightful spread they served him for lunch. My Mum and Dad's meeting was no accident. Nothing in life ever is. It allowed my Mum's family a chance to get to know my Dad, someone they grew to like and respect, especially, the younger siblings, who were extremely fond of him and the stories he told them. When the family christened him *Baboo Achen* and spoke to him only in Malayalam, he had no choice but to learn Malayalam. In fact, he learnt it so well that he was able to conduct the Malayalam services later in Christ Church in Singapore until the Malayalam congregation appointed their own resident pastor from India.

Sometimes, when my Dad stopped by for lunch, he would find my Mum's parents, my *Velliappachan* and *Velliammachy*, visiting. They were beginning to despair that my Mum was going to end up an old maid if she continued to spend her whole life looking after her siblings and their families without a thought for herself. They instinctively liked the young priest who turned up for lunch every Sunday, and they watched as *Baboo Achen* became a household name. The more they watched, the more they liked him and the more convinced they were that he would be a suitable match for their daughter Saramma. Their imagination ran riot as they put on their matchmaking caps and went into a matrimonial huddle.

No spring chickens, my Mum and Dad were busy, hard-working adults, with careers of their own. *Baboo Achen* seemed to get along well with the siblings, and Saramma and *Baboo Achen* seemed comfortable together. Perhaps they could have a life and family of their own. They knew that their daughter's biological clock was ticking and that something had to be done soon, so they quickly went down on their knees to *The One* they always went to when they wanted something fixed. *The One* who had led their family through all the ups and downs of life. They prayed about it and left it to Him, with the occasional nudge. To everyone's delight and relief, the priest and the doctor, cheered on by the entire village that took complete credit for the alliance, agreed to get married across two states despite the differences in language, culture, and background. My Mum held out until my Dad promised never to interfere with her helping her siblings. A promise he honoured right till the end.

My Mum's viewing

When my Dad broke the news to my *Annammal Paatti*, she was ecstatic. She called her friend and travel companion *Ponnammal Paatti* who always accompanied her whenever she travelled by bus or train. The tickets were bought, and a delighted *Annammal Paatti* and her friend boarded the train to go and meet my Mum at the Ettiyapuram government hospital.

Without disclosing her identity as her future mother-in-law, *Annammal Paatti,* draped in a soft silk sari, waited patiently in the queue to meet the lady doctor in her room. When she was led in, *Annammal Paatti* requested my Mum to repair her pendulous earlobes, a trademark of many women in South India who wore chunky gold jewellery. The weight of the solid nuggets of gold, shaped like spheres and cubes, dragged the earlobes down with time, often reaching the clavicle and widening the earhole. Many got them repaired later, when their grandchildren tugged mercilessly at their earlobes, as babies often do, causing jagged tears that bled profusely. My

Mum did a splendid job reconstructing the ear. She excised the redundant part of the earlobe on both sides and sutured her way straight into my *Annammal Paatti's* heart. After the surgery, my *Annammal Paatti* revealed her true identity, and my Mum was flabbergasted. She had thought that the sweet old lady was just another patient. *Baboo Achen's mother?* she gulped. Confused and thrown completely off guard, she desperately tried to rewind the consultation in her mind's eye. *Had she been polite? Had she created a good impression?* The entire consultation was turning into a blurred nightmare. *Oh, dear God, please let it heal well,* she prayed and, fortunately, it did. My *Annammal Paatti* and my Mum did not meet at an official *pennu kaannan* visit. They met as a doctor and patient over a surgical table in Ettiyapuram and remained good friends right to the end.

My *Velliappachan* met my *Annammal Paatti*, and a date was set. My Mum and Dad were married on 23rd April 1936 in the CMS Christ Church in Kodukulanji by the Rev. Alumootil Oommen Mathai. My *Annammal Paatti* crossed the Tamil Nadu-Kerala state border for the first time in her life to attend her son's epic wedding in Kodukulanji.

The Cadavanaltharayil family

When he married my Mum, my Dad's life changed completely and forever. The ebullient *Cadavanaltharayil* family adopted him unconditionally and engulfed him with a love and warmth that transformed him. Overnight, he inherited a family that transcended the blurred lines of language and state. He suddenly found that he was the revered epicentre of a family that doted on him. He had secured a place in their hearts as *Baboo Achen*, the man who loved their *Pengal* well enough to share her with them even after she was married.

Growing up, he had been shunted around between relatives who had taken pity on his blind mother. As the poor relative dependent on their largesse, he was always the outsider watching their happy families from the periphery. Suddenly, he realised that he was not looking in on someone else's family any more. *This was his family,* his very own family. There was no looking back after that. Slowly, he integrated into the *Cadavanaltharayil* family as he transformed from a sombre young man to a charming young son-in-law, an affable brother-in-law, and a loving husband. In short, the young man his in-laws had handpicked to take over as the head of their family. Watching the dynamics in the *Cadavanaltharayil* family, my Dad, who had been separated from his only sister as a kid, realised with a pang what they had missed as siblings.

My Mum's Siblings
The *Cadavanaltharayils* were a typical Syrian Christian family in Central Travancore. Family prayers at dusk and dawn had them singing hymns of praise and thanksgiving in parts and in harmony without a book. My Dad was intrigued by the way the workload was distributed evenly among the siblings with no room for error. Everyone had jobs to do, and grumbling of any kind was unceremoniously squashed. The boys helped in the fields and the girls worked at home, while the elder siblings ran a tight ship with a keen eye on discipline. Basically, they were a happy household with their parents as anchors.

The Tharavad - the ancestral home
Set in a rice field, the *Tharavad* was a red brick house with an open courtyard in the centre that let rain and sunshine in. The monsoon showers beat down on the sloped roof to slide off the red tiles in sheets and splash on the gravel below. A lean-to veranda

wrapped itself almost completely around the house as a thin boundary between the inside and the outside. A rickety wooden staircase perched precariously against a wall led to the attic the *nilavara* where the grain was stored. Above the attic in the space between the attic and the roof, was the loft, the *thattinpuram* where the seeds for the next planting season were dried.

Every square inch of the *Tharavad,* seemed to be occupied by human life at various stages of development, living together in complete harmony. My Dad had never seen so many occupants in any household before. Why his wife's home had more human beings under one roof than some of his churches did!

The Kuli moori - the bathroom

The *kuli moori,* a thatched room close to the well, had no electricity or plumbing. Water was carried in metal buckets from the well to fill a stone tank built in a corner of the bathroom. The girls used the privacy of the bathroom as they attained menarche and went from girl child to little women, while the brothers bathed near the well in their shorts, drawing water from the well. There were no disposable sanitary napkins or tampons. Old clothes were cut up, washed, hung out to dry, and recycled as sanitary napkins. Stoic operations such as these carried out in the still of the night were awkward and vexatious on the red-letter days of a girl's calendar.

The Kakkoos - the toilet

The toilet or *kakkoos* was a makeshift booth in a field a little away from the house. With time and usage, the *kakkoos* moved to hitherto unused spots in the field. It had a deep circular hole at the centre flanked by two flat stones on which the occupant squatted precariously. Covered by rickety *atap* panels made of coconut palm fronds, with no lock on the door, there was no way of knowing if the *kakkoos* was occupied. Though the acoustic enhancement of sound in the *kakkoos* would have given any music auditorium in the world a run for their money, it was recommended that occupants sing at the top of their voice to avoid surprises. The choice of the song did not matter. Nor did it matter if you dropped an octave mid performance, but sing you had to. Sometimes the scorpions lurking in the toilet booth would come alive with the singing and inflict painful bites on the bare feet perched on the stones flanking the hole. As it filled up, the hole was covered, and the *kakkoos* migrated to another part of the field seamlessly. The *kakkoos* was undoubtedly the biggest challenge we faced on holiday in Kerala. All else was fun.

The Adukkala - the kitchen

The *adukkala* overlooking the courtyard where the kids played was the busiest part of the house. Only when the family went to sleep did the kitchen become quiet. Otherwise, it buzzed with a steady traffic of people, smoke, and smells as meals were cooked and served. A wood-fire stove on the eastern side faced the morning sun that flooded in to sanitise the kitchen. Near the entrance facing the courtyard stood a three-legged wooden stool with a large earthen pitcher filled with buttermilk, *moru-vellam*, watered thin and flavoured with green curry leaves, pink shallots, and amber-coloured slivers of ginger: a refreshing cooler for the dusty family that traipsed back in for lunch and a welcome drink for visitors who passed through the house under a banyan tree near a canal.

The Parambu - the compound

The *Cadavanaltharayils* grew most of what they ate in the fields and farmlands that surrounded the *tharavad*. The hardy rhizomes-tapioca *kappa*, sweet potato, and yam—grew all around the house. *Kappa and meen*, the irresistible mashed tapioca and red fish curry combination, is comfort food crafted to draw any Malayalee out of hiding. The land was fertile, and with free-flowing water to irrigate the fields, mangoes, jackfruit, sapotas, custard apples, rose apples, bananas, and guavas grew around the house, together with the bread fruit- a relative of the avocado—a wonder fruit packed with health and nutrition. The kitchen garden had beans, tomatoes, chillies, brinjals, and okra that grew in rows on the ground, while the gourds—ridge and bitter—hung seductively on wooden trellises around the periphery of the patch. The *bilimbi puli,* a pretty tropical tree with clusters of grape-like tart fruit, enhanced the flavour of curries, especially seafood. Fruits like mango and jackfruit were eaten as a vegetable when raw and as a fruit when ripe. A huge tamarind tree sheltered the front porch, while peppercorns grew as creepers on supportive tree trunks. The drumstick tree, the vitamin A–rich *moringa,* grew a safe distance away from the house as it housed a furry white creepy-crawly that could trigger an itchy skin rash. Mercifully, coconut oil—the panacea for most ailments—applied in generous amounts, soothed the irritation.

A little fed a lot
Meals at the *Cadavanaltharayil* house were served on the veranda near the kitchen. A long wooden table with two long benches on either side had the family sitting down in batches to be fed on use-and-throw banana leaves that ended up as biodegradable waste on the compost heap. Mealtimes were nothing short of a miracle - a little certainly seemed to feed a lot. With every passing year the skills of the kitchen team sharpened as necessity became the mother of all culinary inventions, and food continued to appear on the table every

day, and no one went hungry. Thrift was the buzzword, and nothing that reached the *mise-en-place* table was ever wasted. Dumplings made from flour were a smart way of stretching a meal. Bobbing up and down in the aromatic coconut gravy they soaked up all the flavours of the curry to wash down the unpolished rice from the fields.

An older sibling would walk down to the bazaar to buy rainbow-coloured sea fish caught in nets placed the night before. Boisterous vendors would auction baskets overflowing with sardines, whitebaits, and anchovies at the roadside bazaars. Freshwater delicacies like the *karimeen* and the catfish were caught in ponds and canals. As the morning temperatures rose, the fish prices dipped. Once home, well-spiced and cooked with coconut, mango, and the sour *kokum*, the tired fish would come alive as a delicious curry for lunch.

With so many mouths to feed, no part of the fish was ever wasted. The fish head and mango curry, a great favourite with the siblings, was not a curry for the fainthearted. It was a rustic dish that had to be eaten by hand in rumbustious company while sucking noisily at the bones. Much as he enjoyed all the curries his new family served him, there were some dishes that my Dad never took to, like the fish head curry, all of which the adventurous *Cadavanaltharayil* family fell upon with relish.

Sibling no. 14, *Pennamma-kochamma,* affectionately shortened to *Pennacho* by her nephews and nieces, who climbed into her bed in later years to hear the *Cadavanaltharayil* Tales, was incharge of the kitchen. An excellent cook, she rationed out the food that reached the dining table. Sometimes she would catch one of the younger siblings trying to pinch food from the kitchen. Waiting until the hand pushing in through the movable horizontal slats of the window had curled around a piece of fried fish, she would grab the offending hand by the wrist in a vice-like grip and shake it mercilessly until the piece of fish fell back on the plate and the miscreant extricated his hand and ran away squealing in pain.

The Matriarch

As there were no professional caterers, the food for any event in Kodukulanji, including wedding banquets, was cooked at home. The red fish curry, a must at weddings, looked good, tasted good, and could be made weeks ahead in large quantities. With *kokum* as a preservative, the curry never went bad, even during summer. My *Velliammachy* would be invited to supervise the cooking as her culinary skills were legendary. Most of the younger women had cooked for several events and knew the exact amount of spices that went into the curry and could have done it in their sleep. Nevertheless, out of respect, they would bring the spices on a tray to check with my *Velliammachy*. She would inspect the tray, and after a deliberate pause, she would use her right index finger to remove a couple of curry leaves or a couple of peppercorns to one side. The flick of the finger to remove the expendables was deliberate and established her undisputed position as a *POA—a person of authority*—when she held court as the matriarch of the *Cadavanaltharayil* family. Even if you had scanned her until the cows came home, you would not have found even a trace of the tomboy her mother had despaired over.

The famous red fish curry tasted best when slow cooked in a traditional *chatti,* or earthenware pot, over a wood fire: the flavours were enhanced as the alkaline mud pot neutralised the acidity of the food. Sometimes the fish was cooked with an unripe mango or with the green *bilimbi puli,* when the resulting sharp, tart flavours of the curry took finger-licking up a few notches. The bland fish stew, the *fish molee*, on the other hand, was always cooked in coconut milk to tone down the spices for the younger siblings.

Virgin coconut oil, the cooking medium extracted at home from coconut kernels, lasted months at room temperature and did not turn rancid if stored with peppercorns. All the spices for the curries were ground on the *ammi kallu*, the traditional grinding stone. Unfortunately, the *ammi kallu*, a relic in the age of electric mixers, is only a decorative objet d'art in elite landscaped gardens today. Diaspora paid hard cash to carry it as extra baggage to remind themselves of home when they migrated to far and distant lands. Grinding on the *ammi kallu* was a woman's job. It was always done outside the kitchen on the veranda as it left a watery trail when the stone was washed down with water before and after the grind. The cylindrical rolling stone with rounded edges reclining at the head end of the *ammi kallu* was grasped firmly with both hands. With a systematic back-and-forth movement that bulged the biceps and jiggled the breasts in provocative distraction, stone met stone in even strokes. As it gathered momentum, it pulverised everything that came between the rolling pin and the slab, dishing up gustatory delights that modern gadgets and gizmos cannot replicate in taste or texture.

The siblings would wallow in nostalgia when they drooled over the memories of meals made with a bit of this, a bit of that, and a lot of love. The flavours heightened imperceptibly every time the stories were told and retold. Nothing they ever ate later in any corner of the globe compared to the curries served on the veranda of the house under the banyan tree by the canal. An extremely wise lady, my *Velliammachy*, brainwashed her children into enjoying different parts of the bird and fish anatomy, delicacies they fell upon with relish, accepting the adage: *If you don't get what you like, you'd better like what you get!*

My Mum could never pass up the bishop's nose of the chicken in the later years of plenty. She was delighted when she met it again, under rather exotic circumstances, at the roadside food stalls in the *Pasar-malam*, the night markets of Malaysia. Sold as a mind-blowing delicacy known as *ayam paggang*, it comprised the bishop's nose together with all the other discards of the chicken flattened out with a food mallet, grilled on skewers over live charcoal, and served seasoned with mouth-tickling aromatic herbs drizzled with lemon juice. As far as she was concerned, no other part ever matched the taste of the humble coccyx, the bishop's nose of the chicken.

At nightfall, the main hall resembled an Indian railway station platform, with the older girls and the younger siblings sleeping on mats on the floor. The older boys bare chested in shorts, spread themselves outside on the veranda. Eventually, the muffled chatter would turn into an orchestra of snores. Perhaps that is when my *Velliappachan* and *Velliammachy* managed to catch a quiet moment alone?

Get off the train!
When my Mum and Dad were married, my Mum was working as a doctor in Tamil Nadu, having completed the LMP at CMC. Medical education meanwhile had advanced, and Madras Medical College offered a shortened MBBS course to those with an LMP. My Dad thought this was an excellent opportunity for my Mum to upgrade her training, and he offered to sponsor her studies on the double-digit salary he earned as a village priest. They applied and were delighted when she was accepted for the course. This stirred up envious green ripples, as some of my Dad's peers felt he was getting far too ambitious. Some of them marched down to the bishop's house to complain that Baboo, the young priest posted in Sathur, had highfalutin ideas

far beyond his station. He was actually sending his wife, *the Malayalee Lady Doctor*, to pursue her higher studies. If these lofty ideas were not nipped in the bud, they would spread like wildfire, and other young clergy would follow suit doing their own thing to disrupt the work of the diocese. They clucked their disapproval as they stoked the fire with their *tsk-tsk-tsk*. Most men, and the clergy were no different, expected their wives to share the burden of their work, all the while shuffling a few paces behind them. Silently.

Meanwhile, my Mum and Dad had settled down in the compartment of a train bound for Madras. When my Dad looked out of the window, he saw the bishop running on the platform towards their train with his cassock flapping wildly around him. Running alongside were several priests peering into compartments, obviously searching for someone. The bishop spotted my Dad and scrambled into the compartment with his entourage. Huffing and puffing, the bishop threw himself onto the seat next to my Dad. Clueless, my Mum and Dad thought that he had come to see them off. Touched to the core, my Mum offered him a glass of cold water from their mud pot, the *kuja*, that travelled with them on long train journeys. The bishop gulped down the water and started his tirade, wasting no time. *Do get off the train, Baboo,* he said, *working wives interfered with work. The diocese is not interested in them.* He continued to talk about my Mum and her potential to be a troublemaker and a nuisance to the diocese, ignoring her as she sat right in front of him. My Dad, lost no time in standing up to the bishop, pun totally intended, and the priestly sycophants who had accompanied him.

My Lord Bishop, I will get off the train if you order me to, My Lord, he said respectfully. He always sounded like an actor from a Shakespearean play when he addressed his bosses, the bishops he worked with. *But I am extremely sorry that I cannot ask my wife to get off the train, My Lord.* He gently reminded the bishop that my Mum was not employed by the diocese and was free to go to Madras and upgrade her training if she wanted to. The compartment, meanwhile, came alive and watched the tax-free entertainment unfurl with growing interest. Some of them were sure that my Dad was running off with my Mum. They thought that the bishop had found out in time and had come to stop them. *They do not look very young,* they speculated amongst themselves. *Maybe she is someone else's wife.* Engrossed in the drama in the carriage, no one noticed that the guard had blown his whistle and waved the green flag. The wheels started moving, and the train slowly started pulling out of the station. With great presence of mind, the bishop jumped up and pulled the red plunger that activated the emergency brake, bringing the train to a grinding halt. Politely and firmly, my Dad stood his ground and disobeyed His Annoyed Holiness. He got off the train with the bishop but refused to let my Mum get off the train.

After the kerfuffle was sorted out, the whistle blew, and my Mum took that fateful journey alone, leaving my Dad behind on the receding platform flanked by a host of officious white cassocks, to face the music and deal with an irate cleric, his mitre, and his staff. My Dad had ruffled senior clerical feathers, and as a marked man, he was assigned hardship postings far from his wife. This did not bother him in the slightest. He stood his ground, determined that his wife should finish her training, come what may. What they did not know was that he could be painfully stubborn when provoked. Meanwhile, Stephen Neil, the bishop of the neighbouring diocese, who was rather fond of my Dad and I suspect secretly admired his spunk, sent word to tell him that Singapore needed a pastor.

Dear Baboo, the letter read, *There is a position for a resident priest in a Tamil-speaking congregation in Singapore. Why don't you take up this challenge while your wife finishes her studies?*

Regards,
+ Stephen

He gently persuaded my Dad to accept the assignment, by which time His Neighbouring Holiness would have retired, and my Mum would have completed her training and be able to join him in Singapore. When my Dad sailed for Singapore, leaving my Mum in medical college, he had no idea that it would be many long and weary years before he could return to India. They had no clue that a global world war would separate them for years leaving them stranded and incommunicado on either side of the Indian Ocean.

PART 2

Singapore: Pre- and post-war | Christ Church | The Parsonage | The Singapore Siblings | Diaspora | The Indian Holidays

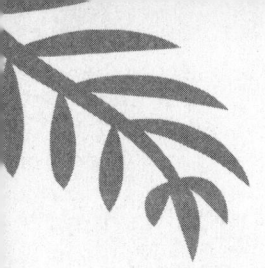

The war years

I did not need a whole village to raise me, I had Christ Church. To understand the impact Christ Church had on my life I will need to take you down the years that my Dad spent in Singapore and made history by being the longest serving pastor of Christ Church when he completed 31 years as their *Pathriyar*. I will need you to understand how Christ Church was his brainchild. His whole life. And ours.

Sir Stamford Raffles discovered Singapore in 1819. Subsequently, people from all over the world flocked to populate the tiny cosmopolitan island, where cultures and races met and lived peacefully. Christians of all denominations, languages, and races worshipped together at the St Andrews Cathedral, founded in 1830. As the services were in English, the migrants who even dreamt in their own language found the English services alien. Religious worship, to be meaningful, has to be in the language you learned on your mother's knee - your mother tongue.

The Tamil migrants, who had ventured out alone to seek employment in an unknown land, were homesick young and old men. They yearned for their homes, their families, and

India, the land of their birth. They were used to hearing the Bible read out in *Tamizh* while they sat cross-legged on the ground. The sermon by an expatriate in English went over their heads, even as they missed singing their devotional *keerthana*s or lyrics to Carnatic ragas. The Chinese migrants too preferred to worship in their mother tongue. St Peter's Church was established on Stamford Road in 1875 in response to the need of the different ethnic groups. This was a time-share home church for the non–English speaking congregations that grew from the St Andrew's Anglican Cathedral. Time-share, a system by which dedicated time slots were allotted to the different congregations, seemed like a solution for a while when the Tamil congregation at St Peter's Church was small and compliant. However, as the congregations grew, there was a rush for convenient slots available for services and time-share was no longer a comfortable option. Slowly, the ethnic congregations moved to their own church buildings, and the Tamil congregation was delighted that it did not have to queue up to worship in *Tamizh*. Before he retired, my Dad's predecessor, Rev. Canon CD Gnanamani, had bought 58,000 square feet of open land at the junction of Dorset Road and Keng Lee Road. A gifted musician, he drew up the plans for a church the Anglican Tamil congregation could use as a place of worship. My Dad succeeded Canon Gnanamani as the incumbent priest in charge of the Tamil congregation when the foundation stone for Christ Church was laid at No. 1 Dorset Road on St Luke's Day, 18th October 1940, by the Rt Rev. BC Roberts, the Bishop of Singapore and Malaya. This was an act of faith in a world whispering of war, when building churches was definitely not a priority. I later learned that whenever my Dad laid the foundation stone for any new building or extension, there was often very little money in his pocket or in the bank to start any construction, though no one would have thought so seeing his demeanour of unshakable confidence. He placed his faith and trust in *The One*, who had blessed him in innumerable ways that could not be recalled, and the money for the construction always flowed in as easily as his prayers.

Alone in a foreign country without his wife and family, my Dad worked tirelessly to raise funds and supervise the construction of the church as it came up, brick by brick. On the eve of Palm Sunday, 5th April 1941, Christ Church was dedicated by the Venerable Graham White, the Archdeacon of Singapore who was also the Commissary of the Archbishop of Canterbury. Christ Church was the home church for the Anglican congregations of the Tamils, the Malayalees, the Telegus, and the Hindi-speaking people, mainly the Punjabis who fought with the British Army. My Dad conducted services at different times for them, with the help of lay preachers and catechists. For a while, the Orthodox Jacobites too used Christ Church until they procured their own premises.

I think the congregation that my Dad enjoyed the most was the Hindi-speaking group. They were the smallest of the congregations, but if you stood outside and listened to them sing, you would have thought that every pew in the church was occupied and overflowing. They praised God with unparalleled enthusiasm. Led by their leader *Danbath*, they would arrive for service in *mufti*, sporting their colourful headgear, the *pagadi*s, while drumming on their *dholak*s and singing at the top of their voices. When they came to church, they sang and danced with sheer joy. No war was going to get their spirits down! Eventually, the Punjabi congregation dwindled, when most of them moved with their contingents to serve overseas, leaving my Dad with the memories of a warm, happy, unforgettable congregation he felt blessed to have served.

Mr and Mrs Sam Williams and their daughter, Pearl, lived at the parsonage with my Dad during the war years. My Dad kept the church and parsonage open 24×7 so that people needing shelter and food could walk in at any time. Everyone shared whatever they had and no one was turned away. Thanks to the ingenuity of the Punjabis of the Hindustani congregation, who were robust agriculturists, every square inch of land around the church and the parsonage was converted into patches that grew food. Their green fingers could make hard rocks sprout, and tapioca and banana grew in abundance during the war years in the Christ Church compound. The food they planted was not for them as they lived in the British Army barracks and had all their meals served hot and on time. Singularly selfless, these born farmers tilled and tended the land for all the other Christ Church congregations who needed it. God bless their generous hearts!

Christ Church bombed

The British had installed an anti-aircraft gun in the Christ Church compound. The anti-aircraft gun gave the members of the congregation a false sense of security. They did not think that the Japanese Army would bomb a church on holy ground. During fierce shelling, they would crowd to hide for hours in the trenches around the church. Huddled in pathetic groups, hungry and too weary to run, they longed for a word of comfort and a familiar face. If they had to die in the bombing, what better place to die than in the church compound? The silver cross at the altar and the anti-aircraft gun in the compound were all the protection they needed. Or so they thought.

My Dad celebrated the Holy Eucharist every day of his life, all his life. He believed that any member of his congregation should be able to walk into the church any day of the year to celebrate a birthday, an anniversary, anything at all, or to receive Holy Communion. Some days he was the only one in the church. That never stopped him from reading the order of service from start to finish or from having Holy Communion on his own. Often, when he turned around mid-service, there would be a couple of congregation members who had walked in late. No one ever went away disappointed that Christ Church was closed even during the perilous days of war.

By February 1942, the British troops were forced to retreat, as the front line of the Japanese Army was moving closer to the heart of the city after crossing the causeway connecting Malaya and Singapore. As the Japanese troops advanced over Bukit Timah, street fighting broke out all over Newton Circus, which was only a stone's throw away from the parsonage in Keng Lee Road and dangerously close to Christ Church on Dorset Road. On 11th February 1942, a few months after the dedication, Christ Church suffered colossal damage from an advancing attack that lasted almost three days. The anti-aircraft gun, a vital target in the church compound, was bombed, and Christ Church suffered a direct hit in which the entire roof of the sanctuary collapsed and the church caught fire. Mercifully, no one was killed as no one was inside at the time. That was the only day my Dad had been persuaded not to open the church. The British admitted defeat and left the island to the Japanese Empire from 1942 to 1945, until the bombing of Hiroshima and Nagasaki.

As news of the bombing of the anti-aircraft gun in the church compound spread, the devastated members of the different congregations rushed to assess the damage their beautiful church, just a few months old and built with blood and sweat, had suffered. They gasped in horror when they saw that the sanctuary had caved in, destroying the altar. The silver cross, the emblem of their faith, lay buried under the rubble. My Dad and his inconsolable congregation members wept in huddles around the ruins as they struggled with the carnage. With trembling hands, they pulled out the silver cross, painfully conscious of the unexploded shells that lay treacherously around them. The candle dampers at the altar had marks of shrapnel until they were changed many years later. The loyal congregation members cleaned out the church, rearranged the pews, and assembled a makeshift altar near the front at the entrance of the church as the sanctuary and altar were declared unsafe. Many churches taken over by the Japanese as warehouses for artillery and supplies were later returned with strict instructions that preaching of any kind was not allowed and only dry bread and water could be used as sacraments at the Holy Eucharist. Restoration of the roof was possible only after the surrender of the Japanese on 12th September 1945 when a sympathetic Hindu gentleman, a stranger from a different faith who wished to remain anonymous, made a generous donation, in the days when money and resources were hard to come by, to replace all the tiles on the roof.

Bonding between bombs

The Japanese installed a machine gun in the parsonage compound and converted it into a temporary garrison for their soldiers. When my Dad and all those who had sought refuge in the parsonage were evacuated, they moved to the Lanka Dispensary at No. 42 Serangoon Road until they were allowed back in the parsonage. Dr KP Pathy, a close friend of my Dad who ran the Lanka Dispensary, lived upstairs with his sons Durai, Mylan, Jambunathan, and Boopalan. They opened their home, slept on the floor, and shared their meals out of a single pot with the congregation members from Christ Church.

Bonding in adverse conditions, with bombs exploding around them, they forged friendships that survived generations, during and after the war years. With time my Dad became a familiar figure to the Japanese soldiers who patrolled the streets. They were quite used to him coming and going as he pleased with his dusty cassock flapping loosely over his bony frame. My Dad moved fearlessly on the only mode of transport he had, a ladies bicycle, through the smoke and grime filled ruins, tending to the sick, the dying, and the dead.

The fierce and often relentless shelling resulted in loss of life and limb in tragic episodes. Many of the Christ Church members were wounded and many carried painful shrapnel well into their sunset years as souvenirs of the war, along with the nightmares that never seemed to leave them. Asleep or awake, the screams of loved ones dying slowly and painfully beside them as they watched helplessly haunted them. The horrendous aftermath of the bombings kept my Dad busy. The dismembered remnants of humanity had to be buried, sometimes in crude wooden coffins and sometimes directly into jagged holes in the earth when token pieces of anatomy were all they had left to gather for burial. My Dad would help dig the graves and lower the dead into the silent echoes of a senseless death with prayers from his almanac.

His work kept him so busy that he had scant time to miss my Mum, his mother, or the *Cadavanaltharayil* family he had left behind in India. Only when he crawled back home to the stark parsonage that served as a garrison for the Japanese soldiers did he feel lonely or homesick. Most days he was too exhausted to think or feel anything. He just crashed onto the hard, wooden bed he slept on without a mattress, waking up the next day to a routine that was just as bleak as it was repetitive. During the Japanese occupation, my Dad was everywhere.

The Japanese soldiers never stopped him from doing his rounds of the congregations under his care and he was never denied access anywhere. He even managed to enter the stench-filled prisons. At the Changi jail, he met the archdeacon, the Venerable Graham White, who had consecrated Christ Church and conducted the dedication service a short while before it was bombed. The archdeacon and his wife had been detained as British POWs, prisoners of war. They both died in prison, but not before they nurtured a magnificent ministry there. My Mum's maternal uncle, MM John, who served in the postal services of Singapore, was captured and, like so many other officers, was held as a POW in Changi. Later, when he succumbed to his injuries, my Dad claimed his body and buried him at the war cemetery at Kranji with the help of the Army chaplain.

When the incumbent Bishop of Singapore, the Rt Rev. JL Wilson, was interned in Changi jail, my Dad was appointed the Bishop's Commissary for *Tamizh* work in the Diocese of Singapore and Malaya. This meant that he travelled extensively over the length and breadth of Malaya to the rubber plantations, where the Christian Tamil migrants worked. This was a link that Christ Church cherished until the Diocese of Singapore and Malaya split after the countries attained independence. My Dad would repeat these wartime stories to me when I was growing up. Charged, his eyes would light up as the adrenaline flowed and he relived the uncertainties, danger, and challenges of the Japanese occupation. His calling as a priest was the only thing that kept him alive during the war. Although I listened to all the stories he told me the many times he repeated them, I doubt if the gravity of the wartime perils meant much to me, a post-war child growing up in peace with no fear or hunger or want.

I just wish I had listened better so that I could tell you the wartime stories he shared of a horrific event, long lost to the world.

Christ Church

The Christ Church congregation was my extended family, and all my growing up memories are linked with the members of the congregation who were so much a part of our lives, some more than others. The relationships we forged in Christ Church fell into an uncategorised slot with no shared DNA, definitely more than friends, and just short of family. As the *Pathriyar's* daughter, I seemed to belong to all of them. Actually, all the kids in the Christ Church family belonged to everyone in the congregation.

Perhaps there was an ethnic slant to this. As a race we were a minority in Singapore and self-preservation was as vital as living and breathing. If something needed correcting, it was done tactfully and on time. If anything needed reporting, the parents would learn about it, more often sooner rather than later. The congregation felt responsible for all the Christ Church kids in a caring and protective way. A mother who migrated overseas told my Dad on one of her visits to Singapore that what she missed most was the protective cordon the congregation of Christ Church cast around all the kids. All the Christ Church kids belonged to the church. Monday to Friday we went to school. On Saturday we had choir practice and on Sunday morning we went to the 8 am service and to Sunday school after that.

Socialising with the opposite sex happened only within the church compound, during church picnics and carol rounds, monitored by every watchful parental eye on site. An Indian boy taking an Indian girl out was likely to go broke as her entire family would tag along as chaperones on their dates. Fatigued, many Indian boys returned to India to seek suitable Indian brides as the effort of courting Indian girls in the Singapore of the 1950s was far too exhausting.

A Sunday at Christ Church

If I am in Singapore on a Sunday morning, I am picked up for the 8 am service at Christ Church by Edwin and Glory Barnabas, Christ Church kids I grew up with. Seated inside, I am swept on an emotional journey down memory lane. A tryst with the past, where familiar faces and voices reach out to greet me and transport me to a safe, happy, and uncomplicated recess of my mind.

I sit there in the present, in the cool comfort of the air conditioning that shuts out the noises from the street, digital acoustics, a screen displaying the hymns as they are sung in real time and a tiled altar, even as my mind wanders back to the memories that leap out at me.

> *I see the doors of the church flung wide open, allowing the street noises in to compete with the noisy fans swirling from the beams above. I see Davis Thatha, everyone's favourite churchwarden, in his white jacket, welcoming everyone at the front door with his kind eyes and warm smile. I see him hand out dog-eared 'pamalai hymnals' and prayer books. I see his pockets bulging with candy for us, the kids who flock to him after the service. I see the congregation split right down the centre by aisle and gender, with the men on the left and the women on the right. I see the regulars seated in the pews they occupied all their lives. If I reach out, I can almost touch my Mum as she sits in the fourth row next to the aisle with her sari pallu*

pinned on her left shoulder and spread out to cover her head. I see Mrs Beebee hit the keys of the organ for the invocation, a signal for the congregation to stand up. I hear my Dad's voice, sans microphone, boom out, 'Jebam panna kadavom. Let us pray,' from the back of the church. I look back to see Isaac Catherasu in his white cassock as cross-bearer, leading the assembled choir in ascending order of height. I hear Mylan Annan's beautiful baritone singing the magical part Nee Vazgha Vazhga as only he could, to the hymn 'All people that on earth do dwell'. I see the choir in short white tunics worn over their street clothes walking in. I see my best friend, Evelyn, walking in next to me, bonded as partners in crime and sisters from different mothers. She is taller than me and she hunches, ever so slightly, so that we are not separated from each other. I see Uncle PV Samuel, our choirmaster, walk behind the kids he trains every Saturday. I see my Dad at the end of the procession going up to the altar and turning around to face the congregation.

These images are so vivid that I cannot believe that several decades have passed. I cannot believe that these are just memories from the past. It seems that it was just a few Sundays ago that we flocked to Christ Church. Where on earth have the years gone?

Coming back to the present, I see my friend David Samuel lead the choir as his father, Uncle PV Samuel, did when we were kids. I stand up and turn to smile at a sea of faces known and unknown when the incumbent pastor introduces me as Canon Baboo's daughter. The number of familiar faces has dwindled through the years, but there is always an inexplicable feeling of warmth that washes over me as they welcome me back to Christ Church—a homecoming, a feeling I pack away and treasure until the next time.

Ashish, our elder grandson, accompanied me on one of my trips to Singapore. Barely seven, he stood up, innocent but supremely confident, when the pastor introduced him as Canon Baboo's great-grandson. Turning around in a panoramic sweep, he waved and smiled at the congregation as they clapped for him. I was sure that my heart was going to burst with happiness. Did I imagine it? Or did I just see my Mum and Dad smiling down at the little boy they had never met?

After church, the congregation moves to the canteen of the assembly hall. Over breakfast, I get to meet the old-timers who knew my Mum and Dad and I cherish the anecdotes they share with me—fond memories of their *Pathriyar* and Mrs Baboo—even as I choke over the lump that forms in my throat.

Christ Church Sunday school

Sunday school classes were held in the front pews of the church after the morning service for *the Christ Church kids*. Mrs Beebee and Mrs Eames, the faithful duo, were the glue that held us together every Sunday with colourful stamps as reward for attendance and good behaviour. They taught us Bible stories and hymns from *Golden Bells*. Hymns we sang so often that we knew them by heart and most of the time could sing them without a songbook. Over the weeks leading up to Christmas, the Sunday school practised with great excitement for the nativity play.

Every year I waited in vain to play a significant role in the play, but the glorious role of the Angel Gabriel always eluded me. Marguerita Beebee, a tall graceful ballerina and tap dancer, was the undisputed Angel Gabriel every year. She was everything that I was not. I would look on in mute envy when she appeared on stage wearing a flowing sequined white dress that shimmered under the bright lights as she announced the birth of Christ. A pair of magnificent wings that were stitched onto the back of her dress arched majestically behind her. Wings she could spread at will by pulling at a pair of ribbons attached to her waist. A tiara sat on top of the ringlets that crowned her head as she flitted across the stage, waving a wand. A trained ballerina, she would pirouette on her toes and glide across the stage – here, there, and everywhere. She was an angel and a fairy rolled into one, the epitome of grace. Everything that I wanted to be!

One year, I remember, I was a goat again and did not even have a costume to dignify my hoofed status. All I had was a white bed sheet that covered me with *GOAT* written in capitals with a blue marker. I was mortified. I crouched in front of the wooden stable on all fours and tried not to scowl. As instructed, I raised my head periodically to *Baaaaaaaaaaaaa*. My Mum and Dad did absolutely nothing! They just told me not to sulk. Disciples of tough love, they were pleased that I had not been indulged in any way. I sometimes wonder if they rigged the casting so that I would not grow up expecting favours from anyone. The appreciative noises that people made over my stellar performance as a domestic goat, in the life and times of Christ, did not appease me in the slightest. One year as one of the Three Kings, I had a crown on my head and one of my Mum's beautiful purple and gold saris draped around me and belted at the waist. I carried my Mum's carved Kashmiri box as myrrh, one of the gifts of the Magi, and I even had a piece of dialogue to deliver that did not go *Baaaaaaaaaaaaa*. I was a happy king who was not a goat!

Christ Church weddings

Marriages in Christ Church, which were held on Saturday afternoons, were a perfect fusion of East and West. The bride, in a gold and cream Benares silk sari and trailing veil, entered on her father's arm as the organ played *Here Comes the Bride*. Bridesmaids, often wearing saris for the first time, and flower girls in frilly frocks and stiff cancan petticoats, carrying little wicker baskets with flowers, would hold up the veil, tripping over their squeaky new shoes. The nervous bridegroom and the best man, in brand new suits, would wait at the altar with sweaty palms, never looking back. The wedding services usually went off without a hitch. Only once did someone in the congregation pipe up an objection when my Dad read out the bit urging people *to speak now or forever remain silent*. The miscreant, jilted by the bride, was determined to mess up the wedding if he could not have the girl he loved. He was gagged and bundled out swiftly by the bride's brothers, bouncers for the occasion, and was not seen or heard for the rest of the ceremony.

    The wedding service and hymns were either in English or *Tamizh*. The lyrics set to Carnatic music, however, were always in *Tamizh*. Wedding rings were exchanged as the wedding vows were repeated, and the veil would be lifted off the face of the bride so that the bridegroom could tie the *mangalsutra*, or *thaali*, around the bride's neck before they were pronounced man and wife. What was left out was the part where the priest said, *You may now kiss the bride*. That would have been too much for the Indian community of colonial Singapore. They would have been shocked out of their wits at any public display of affection, especially on hallowed ground. Romance was allowed only in Indian films with couples skipping around trees, singing duets like a pair of Siamang monkeys, while roses bobbed together in the frame, and bees hummed suggestively in pairs. That was acceptable on celluloid but definitely not in church, and certainly not in Christ Church! When the newlyweds walked down the aisle, arm in arm, to a resounding rendition of the Mendelsohn's *Wedding March*, the congregation would gleefully pelt the couple and each other with confetti passed down the pews. No one ever worked out when or how the East met the West in the Tamil Anglican congregation of Christ Church in Singapore.

The wedding reception was held in the assembly hall next door. A live band played a mix of Indian film music and western pop songs, while the lead singer, Wilson David, an Elvis Presley look-alike in shiny tights, dark glasses, and tutored sideburns, belted out popular film songs in English, Tamil, and Hindi over the microphone in his lovely baritone with all the right moves to groove. The bride and the groom, meanwhile, would go for a drive in a car decorated with flowers, ribbons, and bows. After the official portraits at the photo studio in town and a change of clothes, they would return to appear on stage with the bride in a red and gold Kancheepuram silk sari. Meanwhile the crowd, would have sweated puddles while they waited in heavy silks, wearing every piece of jewellery they possessed.

Youngsters would wait at the entrance with ornamental silver sprinklers and gleefully slosh the guests with rose water to refresh them. On a table there would be a silver bowl with sandalwood paste. Guests would dip the index and middle fingers of their right hand gingerly into the sandalwood paste and take a little to smear in the hollow of their throat and inhale the familiar Indian flavours. Everyone loved the nostalgia of the Indian weddings at Christ Church when everything was kept as ethnic and Indian as possible on a cosmopolitan colonial island.

Somewhere in the crowd sat a VIP who was invited to every Indian wedding regardless of who married whom. The Indian ladies' tailor was a diminutive man in white pants and a full-sleeved white shirt with gold cufflinks. He enjoyed a privileged status with the Indian ladies of Singapore as he had their vital statistics written down against their names in an A4 size notebook in his shop. Though highly temperamental, he was humoured by everyone as he was, quite often, the only Indian ladies' tailor for miles around and in high demand. Sari blouses stitched to perfection and delivered on time were absolute essentials to match every new sari bought. No one dared to rub him up the wrong way in case he ruined the new blouses. The Indian ladies' tailor, certainly a VIP in his own right, was labelled fragile, handled with care, and placed just a few inches away from the high table.

The MC, the master of ceremonies, usually the bride's uncle dressed in a suit and bow tie, would introduce the newlyweds and their families. He would urge everyone to raise their thimbles of wine and join him in a toast to the bride and groom. The nervous bridegroom would respond with a thank you speech and mumble *My wife and I* publicly for the first time as the guests settled down to a sumptuous high tea with sandwiches, flaky curry puffs, cream cakes, ice cream, jelly, and fruit salad. A dummy multi-tiered wedding cake, with only one layer of real cake, would be cut while the photographer and his flash had a field day. Prepacked, even-sized pieces of wedding cake would be distributed among the guests, who would then line up in serpentine queues to bless the couple and bury them with gifts.

For dinner, Haniffa, the popular traditional Muslim cook, would cook mutton biryani in the church compound and serve it with a *brinjal* curry, a sweet raisin chutney, *timun* (or cucumber) pickle, yoghurt (or *raitha*), a ripe banana, ice cream in paper cups, and a sweet *beeda* (the digestive betel nut). The guests hung around in relaxed groups late into the night, greeting old friends and new, surreptitiously checking out children, clothes, and jewellery.

The bridal couple meanwhile retired to the home of the bride or the groom, to a life shared by every relative in town. Sometimes they went on a honeymoon at a later date to Malaya, to a cottage up on the Cameroon Highlands or Frazer's Hill, the popular hill resorts of yesteryears.

Christ Church funerals

As kids, we attended more baptisms and weddings than we did funerals. The only funeral I witnessed as a child was Dr KK Pathy's at the Bidadari Cemetery. When Dr Pathy died, my Dad lost his best friend. Every evening, he would walk from his home to ours to spend time with my Dad. Sipping their tea on the veranda, the two men who had survived the Japanese occupation of Singapore and bonded in treacherous times would seek answers from the Bible to Dr Pathy's burning questions about his new faith. They would talk late into the night, long after dusk when the birds came home to roost. Perhaps I was taken to his funeral, because the Pathys were always considered family. Why even his grand-daughter Susie Pathy was named after me! At the cemetery, I watched in horror as the coffin was nailed and lowered into the freshly dug hole in the ground. I could not believe that friends would wilfully throw fistfuls of mud on top of a friend's coffin and walk away.

Christ Church school funfair & fete

My Dad was a visionary. In a smart move, he built a building with three floors next to the school. The ground floor was a school canteen during the week and doubled up as a church hall on Sundays for the congregation to mix and mingle after the service. The top floor held the science labs, while the middle floor, built as an auditorium, opened up for wedding receptions and other events, securing a steady income that changed the financial profile of the church and school. The steady revenue allowed Christ Church to remain fiercely independent as a church for the *Tamizh*-speaking Anglican Christians in Singapore. When my Dad laid the foundation stone for the Christ Church school, he stepped onto the first rung of a ladder he could not see, in a leap of faith. Like always, the funds flowed in response to prayers with a little help from the annual fundraiser, the school funfair.

The sombre Christ Church compound was quite unrecognisable on funfair days, with colourful bunting wafting in the breeze, turning it into a festive space. The DJ played popular radio tunes on air and accepted requests and dedications of love with cryptic messages studiously omitting names. The proceeds of the sale earmarked for the Building Fund came from the stalls of food, games, books, and clothes. My Mum ran a mega-stall where she always had an interesting array of bric-a-brac for sale; anything from the kitchen sink to her legendary fish pickle could jostle for space on her shelves.

In addition to the stalls, there were guessing games—*Guess the weight of the cake, Guess the number of sweets in a jar*—in which the nearest guess would win a prize. A merry-go-round spinning non-stop from 9 am when the fair opened would creak to a grinding halt only at 6 pm when the fair was declared closed. A popular mix of street food and home fare with *mee hoon, kway teow, rojak, pisang goreng, popiah,* curry puffs, candy floss, *idiappam,* chicken curry, biryani, *roti canai,* and *parotta* meant there was treat for everyone.

Christ Church @ 75

I was delighted when the Christ Church family invited me to attend the 75th anniversary jubilee celebrations on 18th October 2015. Over an extremely emotional evening, I watched the audio-visual presentation of the church's growth over 75 years. Blinking back nostalgic tears when I heard the glowing accolades speakers paid my Dad, I joined the congregation as they thanked God for my Dad's life of service and vision.

The outreach programme of Christ Church started when my Dad built the Epiphany Church in Seletar for a *Tamizh*-speaking congregation who lived on the far side of the island. Seventy-five years later, God's blessings to Christ Church Singapore extend to Pokhara in Nepal. When I heard that the outreach programme had reached the Himalayan peaks of Pokhara, my cup overflowed as I recalled the time that Sam and I had worked in the region many years ago. Never in my wildest dreams did I ever imagine that I would hear a Christ Church youth group sing with youngsters in Nepal. Our lives had run in different orbits, but someone up there had connected the dots for me.

I met Bishop Rennis Ponniah, the first Tamil Anglican Bishop of Singapore. My Dad would have been bursting with pride to see a Christ Church kid dressed in purple, with a pectoral cross, mitre, and cope, carrying a crosier symbolising his role as the Shepherd of the Flock of God at the Anglican Church in Singapore.

God is no man's debtor

Fifty years after my Dad retired and left Singapore, the Christ Church parish deconstructed the old school to raise *The Canon Samuel Baboo Block*, a multi-storeyed landmark with a spectacular blue cross visible for miles around, in memory of my Dad and his selfless service. A sound business module with floors of office space for rent, it assures the church financial stability for years to come.

The Epiphany Church in Seletar simultaneously deconstructed the modest church building erected in 1965 by my Dad for a magnificent multi-storeyed building for the church with multiple halls, one of which was named after my Dad. Moving with the times, the Epiphany Church is now home to *Tamizh*, Mandarin, and English congregations. Rev. Canon Stephen Asirvatham, the incumbent vicar of Christ Church who grew up in the Epiphany Church, shared precious memories of my Dad with me. The unbelievably generous gesture of honouring my Dad's memory, when most people would have forgotten him, took my breath away. It reaffirmed my belief in a faithful God who is neither blind nor deaf. He sees. He hears. He is no man's debtor. He rewards in His time.

Diaspora in Singapore

My Dad never surrendered his Indian passport. Even though Singapore was flooded with state-of-the-art technology, he would install Usha fans made in India in the parsonage despite the paucity of spare parts as he truly believed in the adage *Be Indian, Buy Indian*. My Mum, the practical one in the marriage, became a Singapore citizen when she joined the Government Health Service to work in the Desker Road Dispensary.

When my Mum and Dad started life in Singapore, they took a bit of India with them in a pot, and they guarded it with their lives. When we returned to India on holidays hanging on to all the cultural markers of our ethnicity and Indianness, we looked like freaks as India had moved on with the times. Our clothes bordered on the retro and conservative, as did everything else. Never trimmed, my hair fell down to my knees. Two plaits, tied in coloured ribbons, including green and white to match the St Margaret's school uniform, sprung from the top of my head like two antennae and followed a tedious schedule of its own. I hated the oiling, washing, drying, and combing routine, but my protests made no difference. My hair lived on my head and did whatever my Mum and my aunts wanted it to do.

Dance and music classes

To keep our Indian-ness, we were sent to Bhaskar's Indian dance classes in the Serangoon area to learn the classical form of Indian dance, the *Bharathanatyam*. Preima and Padhma, the elder Doraisamy sisters, and I performed in his cultural show *Shakunthala* as the sequence of the birds in the forest replete with *gunghroo*s on our feet.

For a very brief period, I was enrolled in the ballet classes run by Vernon and Frances Poh. The ballet school was a sprawling bungalow with French windows that looked out onto a lush manicured garden on Keng Lee Road, a few houses away from the parsonage. The room was large and airy and had polished mirrors on all the walls that allowed you to see multiple images of yourself like a kaleidoscope, whichever way you turned. A piano played unobtrusively in the background. The tutu was minimalist, and the pink ballet shoes with their ribbon ties were quite enchanting. Sadly, they moved to new premises, and my pirouettes crashed to a rude halt, ending my dreams of becoming a ballerina and ousting Margareta Beebee as the Angel Gabriel in the Sunday school nativity play.

In addition to the *Bharatanatyam* and the ballet lessons, I was put to the piano and had a violin stuck under my chin for a while, musical skills I never pursued after I left home.

Trust vs instinct

The spouse with the instinct in their marriage, my Mum could suss a person in minutes. If she said that someone was okay, that person usually was. Our male Lhasa Apso, Tiny, tended to agree with her judgment and he never barked at them. When my Mum said that someone was shady, she was almost always right. When Tiny, endorsing my Mum's opinion, tried to nip their heel, Bhaji our Nepali man Friday, would lock him up in another room even as he continued to bark furiously in protest. My Dad, on the other hand, believed that everyone was created in the image of God. He trusted people blindly, got conned completely, and parted with his last dollar willingly. *This Iyah is hopeless,* my Mum would exclaim in exasperation. *How can you trust people like this? Even Tiny knows better!* My Dad was not street-smart, and he may have stepped into every con-puddle he met on the way, but he was the kindest person I have ever known. A gentle giant who laughed out loud, without making a sound.

My Mum's tough love

My Mum was the most selfless human being I have ever known and a study in extremely sharp contrasts. She was your go-to person when you desperately needed help. If you went up to her and told her that you had killed someone, she would rain a few *futtocks on your buttocks* as she called them, with whatever she could lay her hands on: a shoe, a ladle, or a frying pan. She would scold you until your ears smarted before she picked you up and dusted you down. The tears she cried for you would flood her heart but never spill onto her cheeks. Wasting no time, she would then ring the best lawyer in town to defend you. Tough as nails on the outside and soft as cream on the inside, she could have been Wonder Woman, given her intelligence, her talent, her aptitude, and her determination to overcome all the obstacles that she faced hearing-challenged. Courage has many faces, and my Mum's, without a doubt, definitely tops them all.

Missing a selfish bone in her body

There was only one event in my Mum's calendar when we lived in Singapore - the Indian holiday, when we went home to visit our family in India. She returned to Singapore only to start preparing for the next visit. She had a cupboard in her room where she collected everything imaginable for the family. If anyone gave us a present, it walked in a single file, unquestioned, and shut itself into the *Indian Holiday Cupboard* as did every single present we ever received for birthdays, Christmas, New Year, or no-reason-at-all. It also included medical samples, promotional freebies from department stores, and all the *buy one, get one free jamborees* that gripped Singapore the year round. By the time we were finally packed to go to India, everyone in the family was accounted for by name and age, including the unborn babies arriving that year. There was something for everyone.

In addition to her siblings and their families, my Mum had a huge extended family. She never forgot the people who were kind to her when she walked miles to school, barefoot to top the state for her school final exams. Nor did she forget the families who opened their hearts and homes to her when she lived far away from home. My Mum courted thrift to save something for someone—*always* for someone else and never ever for herself. She would return to Singapore with her heart full and her bags empty, all set to start collecting for the next Indian holiday.

My Mum the bargain machine

My Mum was a pro when it came to bargaining. There were no fixed prices in the 1950s, and bargaining was a skill that sharpened with practice. Everyone bargained. It mattered not if you walked, cycled, or alighted from a chauffeur-driven car. My Mum and her regular vendors had a well-rehearsed song-and-dance routine. She would pick up the fruit and ask, *How much?* The shopkeeper would say, *ten dollars*, adding the popular nondescript suffix *lah*. My Mum would start at two dollars while I stood there mortified, pretending that I had nothing to do with this lady, embarrassed that she was actually bargaining as if we did not have money at home. In my mind, only poor people bargained to reduce the price.

Hai ya, How can, lah? Nine dollars okay lah. Very cheap one, lah, he would say. My Mum would put it down and walk away. He would call her back and she would return feigning extreme reluctance. My Mum would inch her way up, dollar by dollar, and the shopkeeper would climb down, cursing in Chinese. A verbal tango later, they would reach half the pre-bargaining price as seasoned negotiators who met on a regular basis.

My Mum's friends

When Sam and I got married at Christ Church, my Mum invited everyone who had touched our lives in Singapore. The church overflowed with friends, relatives, church members, patients, and VIPs. Along with them, my Mum also welcomed her regular vendors and tradesmen. No one was too small or unimportant in my Mum's eyes. All her regulars were invited to her daughter's wedding and all of them arrived to grace the occasion. Young members of the family were assigned to usher them in when they arrived, with strict instructions to make them feel at home. The goldsmith who had pierced my ears was there. Mr Govindaswamy Pillai, who had retailed all the nylex saris that I wore to medical college, was there. The Chinese shop owner, my Mum's bargain partner, was there. The *appam* person, the shy cross-dresser with kind eyes who made fluffy *appams*, was there clutching confetti. Even the butcher from the Tekah Market was there: the protagonist in the threats, *Susie, we'll marry you off to the butcher if you don't eat your vegetables!*

The parsonage

The parsonage at 118 Keng Lee Road no longer exists except in the minds of the people who shared our lives and home. The property now belongs to a business house, Haniffa Textiles, and a modern multi-storeyed house stands in the place of the old Malay house with wooden floors on concrete stilts I remember so dearly.

Our neighbour on our left, Mr D'Souza, a passionate gardener, had a phenomenal collection of orchids that hung on wooden slatted frames under shaded light. The garden was dotted with sprinklers as the epiphytes needed the correct balance of light and moisture to bloom. The parsonage did not have a manicured garden. Our green footprint was the D'Souza garden next door, with its riot of colours - an absolute delight for the eyes!

The house on the right was a Malay longhouse shared by several Malay families. Most of the menfolk, chauffeurs to the expat community in Singapore, were allowed to drive their cars home for lunch, when Keng Lee Road looked like High Street, with its fleet of high-end cars parked bumper to bumper. The spectacular Malay weddings that took place next door were boisterous celebrations that lasted several days. Undulating couples in colourful ethnic *sarong*s, *songkok*s, *kebaya*s, *and baju* *kurong*s swayed seductively all night under the floodlights to the *Ronggeng*, a Javanese dance, even as the kids peeping from the parsonage windows watched, completely mesmerised.

My Mum managed to get five of her siblings to Singapore, and fourteen of the fifty eight cousins grew up together in Singapore, including Shantha, one of the cousins who came from Kerala after her graduation in India to work as a physics lecturer at Stamford College in Singapore. I was delighted to have Shantha live with us in the parsonage, albeit for a short while before I left to study in India. It was like having a big sister of my very own.

Although the siblings and their families lived in different homes eventually, except for sibling no.9, Uncle Philip *Kochuttychaen*, we did everything together and moved like geese, with the parsonage as a pivot. It was anchor to family, friends, and friends of family when they passed through Singapore. Several cousins and babies of the Christ Church congregation were born in the parsonage or in my Mum's maternity hospital, with my Mum as the attending obstetrician to the Indian community.

CJ Philip, Kochuttychaen, sibling no. 7

Kochuttychaen had left his family in Kerala to work in Singapore. Fiercely loyal, he was my Mum's right hand and left, helping her with all the chores in the house and garden when he was off. Saturday mornings would find him wheeling his cycle to Tekah Market with my Mum's shopping list. On Saturday afternoons, World War 3 would erupt in the parsonage when my Mum inspected the shopping laid out on the dining table. *These brinjals are older than I am, Kochutty,* my Mum would declare, poking the veggies disdainfully. *Kochuttychaen*, dusty and tired, from the cycle ride to the market and back, would go ballistic and swear that wild horses would not make him go back to the market ever again. My Mum oblivious to his protests would proceed to decimate everything on the dining table to a paltry 2/10. The following Saturday the cycle would be wheeled quietly out of the car shed and find its way to the market with my Mum's shopping list in *Kochuttychaen's* back pocket. When he returned in the afternoon, the free-for-all-Tekah-Market routine would blow up with no change in intensity or script. By evening, all would be forgotten as *Kochuttychaen* and my Mum buttered and jammed several piles of sandwiches for the coffee break after the Sunday service at Christ Church.

Monday to Friday, *Kochuttychaen's* office pickup would arrive only after I had left for school. As my Mum would have left for work by then, it was his job to see that I ate the bread-and-butter sandwich and the peeled, boiled egg that my Mum left covered on the dining table. Most days, I could quite successfully sneak these out of the house to throw into the canal that ran in front of the parsonage and watch them float out of my life forever. Some days in my rush to get to the Jambatan Merah - the Red Bridge at the end of Keng Lee Road where my Dad would be waiting in his car with the engine running, my aim would be wonky and the food would miss the canal and land on the grassy verge by its side. *Kochuttychaen's* trained eye would spot it on his way to work and he would pick it up as Exhibit A for my Mum when she returned from work. Once, I stuffed peeled hard-boiled eggs into my school bag to dodge *Kochuttychaen*; much to my consternation, the smell of rotten eggs and hydrogen sulphide caught me out in the classroom. Whenever I see boiled eggs, I think of the mishaps mine had in the parsonage.

Kochuttychaen was the penultimate disciplinarian for the cousins who grew up in Singapore. No one knew when this honour was conferred, nor did it matter whose child you were. When he said, *Jump*, we merely asked, *How high?* He went to church only to record every fidget and scuffle that transpired between his nephews and nieces. Only when we became adults did we realise that he loved us all so much and so well, he was willing to be the *sergeant major* in our lives. We never appreciated him enough until he retired and returned to his family in Kerala. Then we realised that he was quite easily the solid rock and pillar the Singapore siblings and their kids depended upon.

Dr BC John, sibling no. 16, Thambichaen

My Uncle *Thambichaen*, undisputedly my Mum's favourite brother and my godfather, was an integral part of my childhood. As the family doctor, he was consulted for everything. My Mum and Dad never did a thing without consulting him: from changing a fuse, to dealing with an ache in their little toe, or sharing a near-death experience.

I was born claustrophobic with *taphephobia*, the abnormal and persistent fear of being buried alive. It has always been my primal fear and worst nightmare, especially after I read a novel about a man who had been buried alive as *undead buried* and had tried, unsuccessfully, to claw his way out of the coffin. I remember making *Thambichaen* promise that he would check, multiple times if needed, to make sure that I would not end up *undead buried*.

Thambichaen told me, and everyone else in the room, that he would do all that and more. He reassured me that he would make absolutely sure that I was dead. What was more, he was going to fix a bell in my coffin, which would connect to the guard's house near the cemetery gate. If I became alive, I was to ring the bell for the guard, the *Jaga*, to hear. The *Jaga* would then inform *Thambichaen* to come immediately and rescue me. It mattered not that *Thambichaen* was at least thirty-five years older than I was when he made these wild promises and that he lived miles away from the Bidadari Cemetery. I trusted him implicitly. If he said that he was going to install a bell in my coffin to alert the *Jaga* at the cemetery, I had no reason to believe otherwise. I just knew he would.

Gracy kochamma

Gracy kochamma, affectionately shortened to *Gracekocho*, *Thambichaen's* wife, was our favourite aunt whom we adored. She would spoil me silly with all the things I loved from the hawker centre on my sleepovers with my cousins—Soma, Sonny, Shoba, and Sobi—treats that were never entertained at the parsonage. Whenever anyone tells me that I keep a neat home, I mentally thank *Gracy kochamma* as I learned everything just from watching her. She kept her floors so squeaky clean you could eat off them. Her kitchen appliances shone, sans chip or scratch, as if they had been unwrapped from bubble wrap the day before when in reality many of them were at least a few years older than me. One rule she never broke and one that her nieces, her disciples all over the world, follow even if it kills them is *that no trace of a party the night before will see the light of day the next morning.* Even if the last guest left at four in the morning, she would stay up and clear the house. Anyone walking into her kitchen in the morning would find the house spotless, the sink empty and wiped down, smelling of lemon grass, with the countertops gleaming and everything put away neatly.

I do this every night out of habit, as I simply cannot leave a sink of dirty dishes to a maid who may or may not appear for work the next day. The other compulsion to clean up every night before I go to sleep is my fear that if I passed in the night, mourners would walk into a dirty house and that would kill me! *Gracy kochamma* did all the work herself, and visitors to her beautiful home sang her praises. One minute she would be cooking, mopping the floors, or hanging out the laundry and the next minute she would be driving her Mercedes Benz around town or shopping on High Street in a sari from her amazing collection with her diamonds glinting in the sun.

I saw her in many roles: as a wife, a mother, a grandmother, her husband's receptionist in his medical clinic, and an aunt. As graceful as she was accomplished, she was a role model for many of us, someone we all loved dearly.

Aunt Esther, sibling no. 17, My Kunjacha

My Aunt *Kunjacha*, my godmother who sailed with my Mum and me from India, lived with us at the parsonage and shared our lives when I was growing up. She was more than an aunt to me. Twenty years younger than my Mum, she virtually raised me until she got married. The day *Kochuttychaen* introduced PS Mathew, Palliath Samuel Mathew, *Kochunichaen* as a prospective bridegroom for his sister, my seven-year-old world crashed. I was devastated when she agreed to marry him. I thought she belonged only to me as there had been no contenders for her affection until he arrived. I was not impressed when they made me a flower girl in a pretty new dress. Barely glancing at my new shoes, I spent the entire Mar Thoma service howling like a wounded animal, when I was not scowling at the camera.

They came home to the parsonage after the wedding, and I had my revenge all planned. I was going to drown my newly acquired *Kochunichaen*, with the 4711 eau de cologne bottle that was sitting on top of the chest of drawers in the room. Fighting sleep, I waited for him to come into my room. The room that had suddenly turned into theirs, the room where *Kunjacha* had told me all those wonderful bedtime stories. *Where on earth was he going to sleep?* I wondered. Suddenly the door opened and there he was, smiling at me.

I hate you, I hate you, I hate you, I screeched a zillion times as I lunged at him, waving the bottle of cologne. *You can't take her away,* I yelled as hot tears coursed down my crumpled face. The surprise on his face soon turned to amusement as I swung the opened bottle and sloshed it all over the place, missing him almost completely. Some of it drizzled on the sheet, some on the pillow, while most of it fell on the wooden floor. Rushing around like a headless chicken, I tripped on the furniture, slipped on the cologne, and landed flat on my back with my feet unceremoniously up in the air. The part of my plan where he was supposed to leave in a box and I would get my *Kunjacha* back and we would live happily ever after had evaporated with the cologne. Someone had rewritten the script, and nothing proceeded as planned. Suddenly, I realised that *Kochunichaen* and I were not the only ones in the room. The room was full of adults, laughing hysterically. Before I knew it, someone had picked me up, slung me over their shoulder, and carried me out of the room, closing the door in my face.

I was determined to spend the rest of my life hating *Kochunichaen*, but that never happened. He became one of my best friends, a favourite uncle, and the funniest man I have ever known. He turned ordinary events into rib-ticklers. It was not what he said but the way he said it that had you convulsing on the floor. Their marriage was truly a happy blend of companionship and humour between two friends who stayed in love long after their golden wedding anniversary. After four boys of their own, Mohan, Suresh, Soman, and Susheel, they stopped trying for a girl, and I continued to be the daughter they never had. When they retired from Singapore, they left their home on the 9th mile on Bukit Timah, returned to Kerala, and built their home in Trivandrum with chickens, rabbits, dogs, fish, cats, and a beautiful garden with fruit trees. A holiday destination we loved.

Kochunichaen's humour was legendary. One day, when they had visitors for tea, the guests complimented them on their home. *You are so lucky to have a good maid,* they said with a tinge of envy, as good maids were hard to come by in Trivandrum. *Kochunichaen* smiled as he said, *Oh yes, we have an excellent maid. The only problem is that every night, she insists on crawling into bed with me.*

Only seconds later did the visitors realise that he was talking about his wife! I lost a good friend when he passed away. He was easily a well-loved and trusted confidant to all his nephews and nieces, who doted on him.

Ponnamma Anne, sibling no. 19

Ponnamma Anne, my *Aunt Ponnamma*, shortened to *Ponnocho*, the youngest of my Mum's siblings, was the baby of the bunch. Absolutely fearless with loads of spunk and spirit, she would take on the world, charging where angels feared to tread. While studying in Mangalore, she decided to become a nun. A photograph was taken and a letter was sent to the family to say that this would be the last time that they would see her dressed in a sari with flowers in her hair. When they saw her next, she would be dressed in a black habit with her cropped hair hidden under the veil as she was marrying the church. The family flapped and squawked at the thought of the youngest and the prettiest disappearing into the cloisters never to be seen again. *We are not even Catholic,* they wailed. They were up against a formidable Carmelite order of nuns, and a well-thought-out plan was set into motion. Her eldest brother, my Uncle *Chandichaen*, and their maternal uncle hired a taxi from Kerala and went to visit her in Mangalore. Since she could not be persuaded to change her mind, they pretended to give in. *Your happiness means more to us than anything else in the world,* they said in a sad voice. Relieved, my unsuspecting *Ponnocho* walked her eldest brother and uncle to the car for a tearful farewell. As he turned to get into the car, *Chandichaen* swung around without any warning, picked *Ponnocho* up in his arms and dumped her surprised frame into the backseat of the car. *Don't take your foot off the accelerator!* he yelled, as the driver sped across town and state border. *Ponnocho* recovered from the shock and cried all the way, repeatedly reminding *Chandichaen* that he was kidnapping a bride of the church. *Chandichaen's* reply was unprintable. When they reached home, she was under house arrest and her mail to and from the nuns was intercepted by the postmaster, who was an extremely cooperative relative. The family believed that marriage cures most ills, and it was decided that she had to be married off.

Several suitors came and left when she scowled at them. One day, a dashing young man, *John Ramakrishna Pillai, Uncle Johnnychaen*, came to see her. She went in with the tea tray threatening to tell them that she had been kidnapped from the altar en route to becoming a nun and a bride of Christ. She did no such thing as it was love at first sight, ending the saga of the convent, the nuns, and the habit to the enormous relief of the family. Soon after they were married, they were recruited by Emperor Haile Selassie to teach in Ethiopia. Just after Soman John, their son was born, *Johnnychaen* succumbed to a chest injury from a wayward cricket ball on the playing field and died. Utterly alone, with no family to comfort her or even look after the baby, *Ponnocho* left Soman with a neighbour and travelled to Addis Ababa in the hearse to bury *Johnnychaen*. A few weeks later, she arrived with young Soman to stay with us in Singapore. A young and beautiful single parent, she pieced her life together and started teaching at Christ Church School. After a while, the family gently suggested that she remarry. She refused. Eventually, she agreed on two conditions: the person had to be a widower and he would need to accept Soman as his own.

The search was on, and AM Benjamin, Alumootil Mathew Benjamin, *Benjichaen*, came into our lives as a comfortable fit. *Benjichaen's* father was the archdeacon who had solemnised my parent's wedding in Kerala. The families knew each other and everyone was happy. Lizamma Aunty, the principal of St Margaret's School, was *Ponnocho's* best friend and her husband, Georgie Uncle, and *Benjichaen* were tennis partners and buddies. A meeting was arranged in their home in Woodsville, and Soman and I went along as chaperones when *Ponnocho* and *Benjichaenn* met. They got on like a house on fire, and everyone was having such fun at *Lizamma Aunty's* house that no one noticed the clock ticking away. Unfortunately, there were no cell phones in those days to send messages to the siblings waiting anxiously at the parsonage. When Georgie Uncle finally dropped us off at the parsonage, the clock had struck ten, and we found a very grim *Kochuttychaen* hanging over the gate. *Oh my God, Ponnamma,* gasped Georgie Uncle, *your brother has not moved from the gate! Good luck!* He hissed as he hastily backed all the way down Keng Lee Road to Newton Circus, against oncoming traffic, without taking his foot off the pedal.

Ponnocho and *Benjichaen* had four kids of their own: Prakash Mathew, Prasad John, Premilla Elizabeth, and Pradeep Oommen. Their home in Port Dickson, a great holiday destination for us when we were growing up, was filled with good food, boat rides, adventures, and fun. *Ponnocho* was a certified *cordon bleu* cook who conducted cooking classes on Singapore TV. She could whip up fantastic fare from nothing and familiar fare from all things exotic. If there is one lesson that I learned from *Benjichaen* and *Ponnocho*, it is this: every birthday and anniversary is a precious gift from God. They never took any anniversary for granted.

At the age of eighty-two, in the space of eight weeks, *Ponnocho* lost two of her children, her eldest son, Soman, and her youngest son, Oomachan. Once again with remarkable courage and fortitude, she comforted the young widows, and all those around her, including Oomachan's infant son. When *Benjichaen* passed on, she was widowed again and left to nurse a heart full of loving memories. No sooner had she adjusted to life without *Benjichaen*, she suddenly lost her only daughter, Premila. Though her heart broke into a zillion pieces a million times over, never once did she waver in her unshakable faith in God. Courage has many faces, my Aunt *Ponnocho* is definitely one of them.

She was the last of the siblings to leave, and her going was the hardest goodbye that we cousins had to come to terms with. She was the youngest living aunt and our last link to our parent's siblings and spouses. We were bereft when it hit us that *all* the siblings and their spouses had gone. There were no more uncles and aunts left to address us cousins, even the septuagenarians and the octogenarians, by the familiar endearment *molay* and *monay*. How incredibly sad is that?

The B&B on Keng Lee Road

Visitors never stayed in hotels those days, and most of the visiting clergy, including bishops from India, stayed with us in my Dad's study, which doubled up as the guest room. As a child, I would wander in and out of their rooms, delighted that we had visitors. The Christ Church parsonage at 118 Keng Lee Road was not a five-star hotel, but it was warm, welcoming, and came with my Mum's legendary cooking.

A white brick house with a sloping, red-tiled roof that peaked twice to keep the interiors cool, the parsonage was raised on concrete pillars along Malay architecture lines to withstand flooding if the Singapore river ever broke its banks. Set away from the iron gate, the house faced an unkempt garden with snakes that often slithered up the steps and tree branches to get into the house and curl up in the cooler areas. They loved surprising people in the bathrooms. Terrified human beings running out and screeching in various stages of undress, with or without soap in their eyes, really turned them on. Over time, and many snakes later, the space around the parsonage was cemented, leaving a colourful oasis of crotons in the centre.

A five-foot broad trim of earth ran around the perimeter of the compound next to the wall allowing trees, mainly fruit trees, to grow unhindered under *Kochuttychaen's* supervision. In addition to the coconuts and bananas that grew all around the house in plenty, there was a huge *Mata Kuching* tree near the gate, with fruits that resembled a cat's eye. In Malay, *Mata* means eye and *Kuching* means cat. There were jackfruit trees, guava trees, jambu trees, and custard apple trees in the compound. The Malgova mango tree in front of the garage flowered to fruit you could smell from the end of the road. We got to eat them only if *Kochuttychaen* managed to climb the tree and wrap each ripening fruit in a perforated paper bag with a purse string before the squirrels running free on the branches of the tree got to them.

Keng Lee Road and its storm drain ran along a canal of

the Singapore river, stretching from Newton Circus to Christ Church with an intersection at the Jambatan Merah, the busy bridge where nine roads met. Before the river was cleaned up, it served primarily as a channel of waste disposal. After the clean-up, the pong disappeared, and the parsonage's status changed to prime waterfront property.

The chicken coop behind the garage housed the white Leghorns that laid eggs for the parsonage. Mid-November, my Mum and *Kochuttychaen* would bring home a couple of turkeys to fatten up for Christmas. Extremely vicious when they were not roasting in the oven, a rafter of turkeys never attacks adults, but individual turkeys would selectively attack kids. Nauseatingly narcissistic, the turkeys would, when let out, make a beeline for the cars parked in front. Strutting and preening, they would peck at their reflection on the shiny coat of paint on the car, leaving scratch marks that annoyed my Dad, who loved his car. *Those turkeys are not going to live to see Christmas!* he would growl.

Tuppence, the terrier, lived downstairs with *Kochuttychaen* until she grew old and feeble. One morning, when *Kochuttychaen* put out her milk, she never showed up. Heartbroken, he searched everywhere, but she was never found. Tuppence had disappeared. We wondered if she had gone away to die, to spare the family the anguish of saying goodbye. Or, had she just wandered away and lost her way home? Tuppence was sorely missed and never replaced.

The tiffin carrier

Our Burma teak dining table with ivory tusks attached to its carved legs was an ecological disaster. It seated ten comfortably and was almost always full with family or friends of family passing through Singapore. During Lent, the forty days before

Easter every year, the parsonage was declared vegetarian, when only plant forms passed our lips, except for milk, as the jury was still out on whether milk was vegetarian or not. Occasionally, when my Mum was too tired or ill to cook, the yellow enamel floral tiffin carrier parked on top of the kitchen cupboard would be taken down. My Dad, wearing an apologetic look, would furtively sneak the tiffin carrier into his car and drive away to collect a carrier meal. This went totally against the grain as we never ate out except at wedding receptions in the Adelphi Hotel opposite St Andrew's Cathedral. He would drive down to one of the by-lanes near the Kandang Kerbau Maternity Hospital, and hoping that no one had seen him, he would dart into *Kutty's Kerala Mess* for a carrier meal. Only when starvation stared us in the face would the tiffin carrier take a ride in my Dad's car.

Some Sundays, my Dad would make an exception and drive down to the Islamic restaurant for their signature biryani dish. On Sundays, unless I am gagged and tied to the top of a tree, like Cacofonix in the Asterix comic series, I could be found crafting a biryani fuelled by my memories of the Islamic Restaurant Biriani – a culinary pastime I enjoy immensely. Much, much later, my Mum and Dad would pick up takeaway food from the hawker centre in Newton Circus, again very apologetically, when the dictum *No food from outside* slowly changed to *Takeaways allowed*. Only when they were older with no domestic house help did they succumb to the changes around them.

My Dad and his car

My Dad loved driving more than anything else in the world and looked after his car as if it was a baby, tending to every squeak and scratch. The mild-mannered *Pathriyar* transformed behind the wheel when he watched pedestrians jaywalking and disrupting traffic. I have seen him annoyed, even angry, but in all my life, I have never heard him use foul language. The exasperated expletives that tumbled out of my Dad belonged entirely to the animal kingdom. Even his favourite term of abuse, *kazhutha*, donkey in *Tamizh*, sounded like an endearment when he used it. When they retired and returned to Madras, my Dad brought the love of his life, his blue Merc back with him. He was offered ridiculous prices that he chose to ignore when the car rolled out of the ship, but he was indignant when he was asked to pay the clerk a bribe to count the cash he paid as excise duty for the car.

My Mum and her car
My Mum decided to buy a car and be independent. Delighted, my Dad offered to give her lessons. Surviving driving lessons from a spouse is the acid test of a marriage. They would leave the parsonage as friends and return fuming. *I am never ever going in that man's car again;* my Mum would hiss through gritted teeth. *I'll walk if I have to, but I will never get into his car again.* When my Dad said, *Turn left,* my Mum turned right. If he said, *Reverse,* she would accelerate. She drove him up the creek and did the opposite of every command he gave. My Mum went from failing one driving test to another until we stopped hearing anything about it as she continued to drive around with the L-plate and a learner's licence. One day, she came home and announced that she had just passed her driving test. We spluttered as we looked around in surprise. And in guilt. We had no idea that she had taken a driving test. Apparently, she had never stopped and had gone from failing one test to another, enduring the ordeal of appearing and failing all on her own. Finally, as she improved with her hearing aid, they cleared

her and she drove a black Ford Prefect, the only car she ever possessed, with a 388 registration that crawled through traffic, completely oblivious to carnage.

The Indian Holiday

Every two years, my Mum, Dad, and I would sail to India on either *The Rajula* or *The State of Madras*, the passenger ships bound for Madras. For nine glorious days, the three of us spent every waking moment together, floating on the high seas as a family with no extras and no interruptions. Something that was not possible in the parsonage, and I loved it. We would arrive at Keppel Harbour several hours before the ship sailed. Our luggage, a ludicrous mismatch of steel trunks, old suitcases, and hastily stuffed duffel bags bursting with last-minute afterthoughts, carried up the wobbly gangplank by porters, was stashed away in our cabin. My Mum did her packing surreptitiously when my Dad was not around and answered in vague monosyllables when asked what the bags contained. *Kochuttychaen,* her willing accomplice, supervised the loading and storing of the luggage in our cabin. After a carefree spell at sea with the wind in our hair and no land in sight, we would land on terra firma when the haggling with porters and taxi drivers in the heat of Madras would leave us limp. My Dad, who never shopped or bargained in Singapore, was completely out of his depth when he had to deal with the porters and taxis in India. Eventually, one side, my Dad's usually, would wilt in the heat and give in.

The haggling and the hauling would start again at Egmore when we boarded a broad-gauge train to Tuticorin, the railway station closest to Senthiambalam, for a couple of weeks with my *Annammal Paatti* before we set off to Kerala to my Mum's family. My Dad, who lived in his cassock in Singapore, never wore one during our travels in India. He wore colourful Hawaiian half-sleeve shirts that gave him a carefree, *Pathriyar-is-on-holiday* look. Counting our luggage at regular intervals during the journey to see if we had been robbed along the way, my Dad would record the inventory as *x pieces of luggage, plus the kuja = x+1,* the *x* a variable from a dozen to multiples of twelve. The *kuja* was a slender earthenware pot that cooled the potable water we carried with us when we travelled.

Passengers boarding the train would glare at us as inconsiderate space hogs because our luggage blocked the compartment and passageway. *Tsk Tsk Tsk,* they would grumble as they stumbled over our luggage to find their seats. My Mum, looking out of the window, would behave as if she had nothing to do with my Dad or the luggage as he deflected their dirty looks and comments with an apologetic smile from time to time. When passengers alighted, they had to climb all over our luggage with their own held high above their heads. During the overnight journey, my Mum and I slept while my Dad stayed awake to guard the luggage and the *kuja* until we reached Tuticorin, where someone from my *Annammal Paatti's* village would be waiting to take our luggage, the *kuja*, and the three of us home to a beaming *Annammal Paatti*.

After a few weeks at Senthiambalam with my *Annammal Paatti*, we would leave to visit my Mum's family when my Uncle Chandy, *Chandichaen*—CC John, sibling no. 6—came to Senthiambalam to escort us to Kerala, relieving my Dad of the hassle of dealing with porters, luggage, and the *kuja*.

Crossing the linear state boundary of Tamil Nadu and Kerala as the train sped through the tunnels of the Western Ghats, we watched the countryside change to lush green with every passing town as did the script on the bleached yellow concrete slabs bearing the names of the stations. The checked, coloured lungis, worn full length in Tamil Nadu, changed to white *mundu*s, folded at half-mast in Kerala, even as the language and accents of the vendors at the station shouting *Chai, Kaapi, Chai* changed as they ran up and down on the noisy and crowded platforms. Alighting at Kottarakkara, we climbed the hilly road to Kodukulanji in taxis, creaky shells in comic states of disrepair, some even without glass in the windows. When it rained, we were given umbrellas to unfurl outside the window to dodge the deluge. After a precarious journey uphill, in a taxi held together by prayer, we would reach *Chandichaen's* home in Kodukulanji to a glorious reunion with my Mum's siblings and their families, who would have assembled earlier, to jubilant shouts of *They've come! They've come!*

Santhosham Velliappachan

Cousins are the first set of friends you make in life. As an only child, my cousins were my whole life. With at least thirty or forty of the fifty-eight cousins in *Chandichaen's* house in Kodukulanji, it ran like a summer camp. Their sprawling home looked out onto velvety green paddy fields with a huge fishpond near the gate where multi-coloured fish darted in and out of the water hyacinths. Technically, it was out of bounds for the kids. In reality though, everything happened around the fishpond, when we were not climbing the trees that grew taller with every visit.

Most of the cousins played in groups. My gang of four had Jaya, Babu, Reggie Jnr, and me. Jaya was older than Babu, and she never let him forget it. Babu was a few months older than I, and he never let me forget it. All three of us were older than Reggie Jnr, and we never let him forget it. Age bestowed unquestioned authority among the ranks. Jaya, the ringleader, was a tall and lanky tomboy I adored as her slave in every prank and escapade.

It made no difference if we had watertight alibis miles away from the scene of the crime. Our gang, constantly in and out of trouble, was always the first to be hauled up for questioning.

Sometimes, friends from Singapore visiting India at the same time would come over to visit. That is how Mr Santhosham, a parishioner from Christ Church, came to spend a holiday with us in Kerala. Jaya studied him suspiciously from a distance and decided that he wore dentures. When she shared her discovery with us, Babu pooh-poohed it and said that those most certainly were not dentures. They were his original teeth as they were a dull yellow, almost as if they had aged with him. *Dentures are usually white,* Babu pronounced in a superior voice. A heated argument followed, and it was decided that at night we would check to see if the teeth in question lived in his mouth or in a glass of water by his bedside. We waited until *Santosham Velliappachan* had retired for the night, and when the house was still, we crept out and peered into his room from a window on the veranda. It was dark, and we could not see clearly, except for the moonlight reflected in a glass of water by his bedside. Jaya said she saw the dentures floating in the water. Babu disagreed. *There was nothing in the water!* he scoffed. The argument was getting louder, and as there was no consensus, there was only one way to find out. We put our hands through the bars on the windows, but we could not reach the glass. *We could get my fishing rod,* offered Reggie Jnr in a loud voice. Hushing him, we tiptoed back and found the fishing rod without waking anyone. Reggie Jnr stood on Babu's shoulders and very carefully manoeuvred the fishing rod into the room. After several unsuccessful attempts, he managed to hook the gleaming dentures out, dripping water all over the side table and the floor. Just then, *Santhosham Velliappachan* coughed and spluttered as he turned in his bed. In sheer fright,

Babu dropped Reggie Jnr, and we all ran for cover. Running as fast as his little legs allowed but never relaxing his grip on the dentures, Reggie Jnr ran into the house after us. Going back to the scene of the crime was not an option, so we went off to our dorms to sleep, hoping to replace the dentures in the morning before *Santhosham Velliappachan* got up.

We must have overslept because the next thing I knew, they were shaking us awake. Babu and Reggie Jnr were already getting the third degree when we arrived at the court martial. *The old man from Singapore lost his dentures in the night,* growled the angry elders. *He is wandering around clicking his edentulous jaws, looking for his teeth,* they said. *Enthoru kashtam*! They grilled us. They threatened us. They even waved the *vadi* at us. The *vadi*, a shaved green twig, lived as a linear lie detector in homes that believed that sparing the rod spoilt the child. It would be held in the inquisitor's right hand while some part of the child's body or clothes would be held in the left hand to prevent the child from escaping. Raising it a few feet away from the child, the *vadi* would be brought sharply down in several threatening strokes without actually touching the child because that was all that was needed to get the truth out. If the denials persisted, the *vadi* would land on some part of the child's anatomy, an outstretched hand or a palm clenched in terror, the bum or bare legs, and cause a painful welt.

The menacing *wooooooooosh* sound as the *vadi* cut through the terror in the air would make most kids pee in their pants and for every guarded secret to come tumbling out. Predictably, the *vadi* had a short shelf life. It either broke in use or disappeared, only to be replaced almost immediately by another tender twig from the garden. If the *vadi* was not found and punishment had to be swift, anything handy that the eyes fell on would suffice, be it a ladle, a slipper, or a hairbrush.

Technically, Jaya and I were girls and visitors on holiday, so we had some immunity against the *vadi,* unlike Babu and Reggie Jnr, who lived through encounters with the *vadi* on a daily basis when their mother, my *Aunt Kunjamma*, needed to discipline them. We feigned surprise. *False teeth? Fancy that!* We exclaimed. We lied through our back teeth and fled, not caring that nobody believed us. Eventually, the dentures were found behind the sofa and returned to an extremely grateful *Santhosham Velliappachan.*

A Price on our heads

Mealtimes in *Chandichaen's* home had us cousins eating in batches around the farmhouse table on the veranda. First, the little ones would be fed, then the next batch of little ones, and so on, until all the cousins were fed. The menfolk would sit down for a meal at the dining table in the dining room, and finally, the ladies would have a leisurely meal on the veranda, certainly not before three in the afternoon. My Aunt *Major TA John—Thankamma-kochamma,* affectionately shortened to *Thangocho*, sibling no. 12—retired as a matron in the Indian Army. When she timed her leave with ours, the holidays in Kodukulanji were even more exciting. Her steel trunks contained all sorts of surprises, trinkets, make-up, and a world of sophistication she dished out to the impressionable cousins. During mealtimes, she would walk around the table, place her hand on our heads, and call out a number. This was the dowry our fathers would have to pay to get us married.

The pretty ones who took after her, she claimed, needed only paltry amounts or nothing at all as they were so pretty they would be snatched away. The plain Janes had larger amounts quoted, and the rest of us who did not fit the bill any which way at all, were encouraged to elope as no dowry would be even remotely enough. Beauty of spirit never featured in *Thangocho's* classification!

Chatti-choru

The nostalgic flavours of our childhood, cooked on wood fires in earthen pots, were mind-blowing. One heightened flavour that lingers is *chatti-choru*. Rationed out in the kitchen on a first-come-first-served basis by *Kunjamma-kochamma*, *chatti-choru* is a universal favourite, although it cannot be found in any cookbook. Normally, the earthenware pot in which the curry is cooked has a smattering of fried masala stuck to it, a tragic waste of flavour lost in the wash. Ingenious mothers would throw in a few fistfuls of cooked rice together with curry leaves, salt, and a dollop of ghee to fry in the vessel. The rice, mixed with the leftover masala, turned into an unforgettable, aromatic fried rice, oozing zest, and unbeatable flavour. We would have traded our birthright for a mouthful of *chatti-choru* from *Kunjamma-kochamma*.

The secret was to arrive at the kitchen door before anyone else did. If you beat someone else to it, the *chatti-choru* tasted even better if that was possible. Especially, when savoured slowly in front of every envious eye in sight. We appeared at the kitchen when hungry, oblivious of the organisation that went on behind the scenes for the food that appeared on the table. *Kunjamma-kochamma* opened up her heart and home, making us a loving part of her family. I do not think that she knew the pronoun *ende*, for my or mine. Everything she talked about started with the generous and inclusive pronoun *nammade*, ours. *Our house, our food, nammade everything*. *Kunjamma-kochamma*, a child bride at thirteen, grew up with her mother-in-law, my *Velliammachy*, to become the quintessential *Kodukulanji Ammachy*, the glue that held us together and loved us unconditionally.

The dhobi

On our holidays in Kodukulanji, a human washing machine, the *dhobi*, would set up a launderette in the backyard near the well. The dirty laundry, marked with indelible ink and tied in a bundle, was washed with a bar of soap down at the river and then beaten mercilessly against a rough stone to remove any stubborn stains. After a final rinse with an inky liquid that made whites whiter and colours brighter, the clothes were dipped in starchy rice water drained from cooked rice before they were hung out to dry on clothes lines that seemed to block sunlight for miles, while the watchful *dhobi* stood guard with a stick. Crisp, bone-dry clothes were ironed on a pile of blankets with a cast-iron press filled with live coal. It had no inbuilt thermostat, so temperature regulation came with practice: they sprinkled cold water to cool the iron or packed hot coal to heat it. By nightfall, the ironed clothes formed neat piles on a bench, with no mix-up or loss, while the ingenious cousins found many uses for the discarded charcoal.

Every morning, awakened at 5 am for family prayers, we would sleepwalk to collapse in untidy piles on the floor of the sitting room until we were poked and pinched awake to sing and pray. Prayers over, there would be muffled giggles as some of the cousins found their faces painted with the *dhobi*'s charcoal that had found its way into mischievous hands.

Talentime

During the day we played in groups, and at night the family would gather in the courtyard for an evening of entertainment by the kids. These were impromptu acts of genius that Reggie Senior, a talented elder cousin, choreographed for an extremely appreciative audience. With no gadgets and gizmos, we had to find ways of entertaining ourselves. A favourite encore was the impersonation of the village drunk, *Neythonni* by Reggie Jnr, who staggered about slurring, *Fathersh, mothersh, brothersh, shishtersh, and all othersh*. Sometimes when we ran out of skits, we would enact jokes with a scatological tinge, that would bring the house down. One evening, we did the one about an Indian boy's maiden trip overseas.

Scene 1: After a tender farewell at the airport, Reggie Jnr boards a plane to London, fumbles with his seat, screaming at take-off.

Scene 2: At the hotel, the bellboy Joey asks Reggie Jnr if he wants dinner. A sleepy Reggie Jnr declines. Joey recommends something light, like soup. Reggie Jnr declines again, goes to bed and forgets to lock the door.

Scene 3: Babu, a patient asleep in the next room, needs an enema for an outpatient procedure at the hospital across the road. Disturbed and anxious, he tosses and turns.

Scene 4: The hospital paramedic gets the rooms mixed up, enters Reggie Jnr's room by mistake and does the honours on a jet-lagged Reggie Jnr.

Scene 5: An exhausted Reggie Jnr returns home wan and tired. His buddies ask about his trip. He shakes his head ruefully and says, *If they offer you soup at night, drink it! If you don't take it one way, they will give it the other way!*

The audience collapses into loud claps, cheers.

Canon Simon John Pothen

All of us fifty-eight cousins grew up in a world completely different from the one the siblings described. We multiplied, had families of our own and moved to all the corners of the earth. Unfortunately, we never met as often as we would have loved to. We kept in touch through social media to celebrate marriages, births, and deaths, never forgetting the camaraderie we had shared growing up.

Simon was the only one of my fifty-eight cousins who became an ordained priest like his Dad and mine. The telegram from Calcutta, announcing his birth reached the parsonage on my tenth birthday. Telegrams meant only one of three Ds to my Mum: death, doom, or disaster. She was flummoxed when Sam sent me *I love you* telegrams from the far and distant places he travelled to. She was delighted when the telegram announced that Simon John Pothen had arrived on 15.11.1956. Later as a toddler, Simon, his parents, and younger brother, Philip, still an infant, came for a holiday to Singapore. I got an earful from my Mum when I let Simon fall all the way down the steps of the parsonage on my watch as his babysitter. Mercifully, he was a well-padded, chubby toddler and his surprised screams did not in any way reflect the toss he had taken, one he claimed left him scarred for life.

Simon sang soprano as a child in his Dad's choir. His exceptional voice was discovered, and he went on to cut a record and play five instruments with panache. He won a music scholarship at Oxford before he entered the Anglican Church in England. I met *Simon-the-Dude*, as his brood called him, his lovely wife, Deborah, and their five children, Joshua, Abigail, Beth, Martha, and Noah in Pinner (England), where he served as a parish priest before he moved to Chelmsford Cathedral in Essex as the resident canon to shoulder enormous responsibilities at an incredibly young age. I noticed how comfortably fatherhood sat on his handsome frame as we spent a lovely afternoon playing catch with his kids in their backyard.

Simon spent two unforgettable holidays with us in India, when he brought his eldest daughter, Abigail, and later his younger daughters, Beth and Martha, and their friend Grace to meet their cousins. They were magical weeks of fun, fun and more fun. He would play the piano and we would belt out the oldies. We played noisy board games and dumb charades. Every time he won, he would prance around and gloat that he was the best. He was absolutely hilarious, and we let him win most of the time just to see him perform his victory dance. Our grandkids Ashish and Rohan were delighted to have *Simon Appachan* fly kites with them and roll on the grass. I would tell him all the silly jokes I knew, and he would laugh as if his life depended on it. Driving back to Chennai after visiting Mohan and Becky, our cousins in Pondicherry, we told each other jokes to pass the time. I could have sworn that he laughed non-stop for several kilometres over the joke about the young man from India who was given an enema by mistake.

It was easy to be happy when Simon was around as he was one of the happiest people I have ever met in my life, someone who was so very comfortable in his own skin. When we were not laughing together, we would talk about men and matters, and I was impressed by his understanding of life. An excellent cook, he avidly collected recipes of Indian food to duplicate when he returned home. He took some of my fish pickle back with him despite my disclaimer that I was not responsible if it broke or leaked in his luggage, and if the smell lingered on his clothes for five generations. He shrugged nonchalantly as he clutched the sealed bottles to his broad chest, skipping away like a happy child, to pack his bags. Mercifully, it survived, and he mailed me to say that he was glad that he had taken it despite my misgivings and that he would be back for more.

I never saw him again. A few months later, he wrote to tell me the sad news that he had been given just a few months to live. It knocked my whole world over because my memories were those of a happy, healthy, handsome human being in his prime, a young man who was the life and soul of any party, an unforgettable personality whose aura entered the room before he did. He passed away peacefully on 13th November 2017, two days before his birthday, surrounded by his loving family. Simon has been gone for a long time, but I have never stopped missing him.

PART 3

Retired and Relocated | Madras | Orphaned

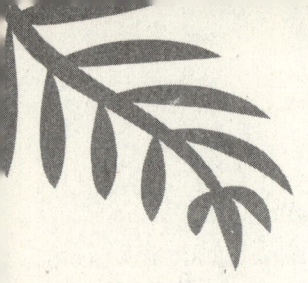

Retired and Relocated

When my Dad retired in 1972, my Mum and Dad were promised a post-retirement job in Malaysia. Unfortunately, it fell through, and they returned to India and settled down in Madras with no definite plans in hand. India had changed in so many ways, and retiring to Madras was a huge challenge. Every passing day made them question the wisdom of their move. Strangers to Madras, they had left behind a lifetime of memories and all things familiar. More importantly, they lost their extended family, the Christ Church congregation, when they landed in Madras.

Bishop Leslie Newbegin, the incumbent Bishop of Madras, was delighted to welcome my Dad and his honorary services to the CSI Diocese of Madras. They were posted to George Town, earlier known as Black Town, to serve at the CSI St Mark's Church. The Anglo-Indian congregation had thinned as most of them had migrated to Australia, leaving a decrepit church compound hemmed in by crowded homes on all sides. Not a popular posting among local pastors, St Mark's Church was threatening to disappear as another lost landmark of Madras. Bishop Newbegin was relieved when my Mum and Dad agreed to look after St Marks while their home was being built in St Thomas Mount. During his tenure, my Dad raised the funds to build a nursery school next to the church and turned the fortunes of the impoverished church marginally, restoring it to a glimmer of its past glory.

When their house was complete, my Mum and Dad moved to St Thomas Mount. The first floor of their house was built as an apartment for rent. Tenants in any part of the world can end up being walking nightmares or relationships made in heaven. My parents struck gold when Vimala and Victor Milner moved in with their kids Sheryl and Sunil to be the only tenant my parents ever had. The Milners became family that stayed upstairs and paid rent. My Dad, in his wisdom, had just one rule for both houses. To eliminate the tittle-tattle that would inevitably lead to misunderstandings between the families, they agreed that no maids, drivers, or other domestic staff were to be shared between upstairs and downstairs. My Dad was a wise old man.

When my Mum had family or guests visiting, Vimala would run down, help her with the cooking, set the table, and run up the steps when the guests appeared. With time when my Mum found it hard to read the inland letters her family sent to her, written in Malayalam, Vimala used to run down and read the letters out loud to my Mum and write the replies. Vimala ended up privy to most of the family's secrets, skeletons, and recognised all the black sheep when they came to visit.

The Milners never ever stepped over the line in all the years they lived upstairs. My Mum and Dad never became Uncle and Aunty or *Appachan* and *Ammachy*. However, when they addressed my Mum and Dad as Rev. Baboo and Mrs Baboo, the respect and love was tangible. They were with my Mum and Dad to the very end. When the ambulance took my Mum on her final journey to Apollo Hospital, Vimala was by her side holding her hand. When my Dad needed his final admission to the Balaji Hospital, it was the Milners who accompanied him. They moved out only when the house was renovated after my Dad and Mum passed on.

My Dad was delighted to help out when the local priests needed him. Sundays would find him driving all over the city to take services in churches in different corners of Madras. If they needed someone to do the odd baptism, wedding, or funeral, he would step in, glad to help out. When I teased him by calling him a *stepney* priest, he would just laugh and tell me that priests never retire, and he was so right.

Sam and his MIL's khus khus

We would visit my Mum and Dad in Madras on holiday from Bhutan and Nepal. Housebound, my Mum was clueless about prices and inflation as she never went shopping. If we bought her anything, we would mark down the price by at least thirty per cent. Even then, she scolded us about wasting money. Sam would try to score brownie points with his mother-in-law by running errands for her and doing everything in his power to make her happy. My Mum and Dad treated him like the son they never had while I watched in amusement, remembering how hard they had tried to break us up in college. People in St Thomas Mount actually thought that he was their son and I the daughter-in-law!

One Sunday, my Mum was halfway through a korma when she realised that she had run out of *khus khus*, the poppy seeds used to thicken the gravy. Unasked, Sam jumped up and offered to go while I watched in utter disbelief. This is the man who would have given me a hundred excuses, in five different languages, if I had asked for *khus khus* on a hot

Sunday afternoon before lunch. He would have questioned the role of *khus khus* in the korma and asked me for evidence-based data to support it. He would have gone on to wonder if all the women in the world cooked with *khus khus* in this day and age. His response would have been pretty predictable, and he may even have declared *khus khus* contraband. He came back a short while later, carrying a large brown paper packet in both hands. My Mum was delighted until she saw the size of the packet. In his outstretched hand was a brown paper packet with five kilos of *khus khus*! For once in her life, my Mum was speechless. She looked down at the package and then up at Sam, hovering expectantly for a mental pat on the back. She looked down again at the package in disbelief and then up again at Sam in horror. She knew that she could not say a word against her dear son-in-law who was only trying to be helpful, but she had to vent her feelings of dismay. She called out to me to complain and possibly scold me on Sam's behalf, but I had escaped into the bathroom to giggle behind closed doors. So, she went looking for my Dad, relaxing in his favourite armchair, watching TV while waiting for lunch.

Iyah, just look at this Psalm, she said, showing him the paper packet. She pronounced Sam as Psalm.

What am I going to do with five kilos of khus khus? She vented on for a while until she realised that my Dad was laughing silently and helplessly. *Khus khus* was not the only thing Sam bought in large quantities for his mother-in-law. He bought her large packs of anything she wanted, to keep her well stocked. With time, she learned to tell him the quantities she wanted, to avoid a *khus khus* repeat. Years later, when we were posted to Bhutan, brilliant poppies leapt out of the flowerbeds at Gidakom Hospital, bobbing in silent laughter. We both turned to each other spontaneously and burst out laughing, remembering another time, another place, and the five kilos of *khus khus* that Sam's mother-in-law must have ploughed through.

What the fish
My Mum made the best fish pickle in the world. She would marinate bite-sized cubes of the fleshy *ikan tenggiri*, from the Tekah Market. The marinated fish was spread out on a large steel tray and placed on a stool in the veranda to dry out before frying. It was my job to see that the pesky birds perched on the wooden rafters of the veranda of the parsonage would not take off with the fish in their beaks. They would squawk in protest, but strangely enough, none of them swooped down for the fish. My Mum swore by a trick to ward off the birds. Around the tray at all four corners, she would place four dried red chillies, and sure enough, no bird came near the plate even though they agitated from above. If the four dried chillies were not in place, the birds swooped down and flew off with the fish.

When my Mum and Dad relocated to Madras, Sam and I were working in the landlocked Himalayas, deprived of the seafood that we fantasised about. My Mum would pickle seer fish (*vanjiram*) from the Saidapet fish market for us to take back along with all the other goodies she made to remind us of hearth and home. The routine was the same. The marinated fish with the four sentinel dried red chillies would be placed on a steel tray on a stool in the veranda of their home in St Thomas Mount. The angry crows protested from the mango tree that spread its branches across the veranda, but not a single one dared swoop down to fly off with the fish. Birds on either side of the Indian Ocean knew that the fish was off-limits if the four sentinel chillies guarded the corners of the tray. When done, my Mum would pack the pickle in a vinegar-washed, sun-dried, empty glass Horlicks bottle, filling it up to the brim with love and care. She would then seal the lid of the bottle with melted wax from candles so that it would not cause an oil leak in our suitcase. Since she had no bubble wrap or cling film, she would wrap the glass bottle carefully in a Kerala towel, a *thorth*, held tightly in place by several rubber bands to act as a buffer to prevent the bottle from breaking en route. Even the faintest leak would have ruined the entire contents of our suitcase.

Your suitcase will smell for five generations if the bottle breaks, she would warn us and laugh when Sam told her that the chances of the pickle reaching home were extremely slim as it would, in all probability, be finished off en route. This act of love did not ever miss a single step every time she made fish pickle, not in all the years I was growing up with her nor when she did it for the last time at the age of eighty when I spent my last holiday with her. My fish pickle is not as good as hers as I do not have the patience to marinate the fish in direct sunlight with the four sentinel, dried red chillies. Nor do I have the magic of her fingers to make ordinary food taste exotic. However, every time I make fish pickle, I remember my Mum, her sentinel dried red chillies, and the pesky crows.

Living with deafness

The world is kind to the blind but cruel to the deaf. No one knows this better than me. I had a grandmother who was blind and a mother who was deaf, and I have seen the differential treatment at close quarters. The blind, are usually treated with sympathy and kindness. People will trip over themselves to help the blind cross the street, not so with the deaf. Deafness echoes with irritation and impatience. The deaf often speak loudly, perhaps to hear themselves. The family, irritated and embarrassed that everything has to be repeated, and repeated loudly, become resentful. Everyone, including the person straining to hear, becomes frustrated. This can destroy relationships unless love and understanding echo in their hearing-challenged world. Hearing aids in the 1950s were bulky and cumbersome monstrosities that often entered the room before the person did. The vain did not go near them and some even feared that they would get electrocuted if they switched them on. My Mum made a few half-hearted attempts at wearing one, but eventually, she gave up the very idea of sound enhancement. *It just makes my deafness louder,* she would say. A statement I still do not understand, but it sounded perfectly reasonable when she said it. If I spoke in my normal voice, she would get irritated when she missed bits of the conversation and say *Speak up, Susie, I can't hear.* If I spoke louder, she would look up quite hurt and ask, *Why are you shouting?* If I retorted something under my breath, she would hear it clearly, especially if I did not want her to. I could never win!

My Dad was the one person in her life who never let her feel handicapped. He would update her on everything, patiently and with much love. Though my Mum was hard of hearing, she and my Dad shared a wonderful relationship, one that many couples, with all their faculties intact, would have envied. What my Mum could not lip-read, my Dad wrote out for her. As she grew older, we used to write on her forearm to read as a mirror image, in reverse. As a child, I would hear them talking in the next room while I was falling asleep, probably updating to bring her up to speed. They were fiercely loyal to one another and touchingly protective. When she could no longer walk outside, she would walk up and down the length of the living room, feeling her way around the room. In the later years, when my Mum started losing her vision, my Dad would never let anyone rearrange the furniture. Everything had to be left exactly the way my Mum remembered it as she faltered in unfamiliar settings.

She used to ask me, when I came home on holidays, if modern science had found a cure for deafness. Her busy home that had sheltered so many over the years suddenly echoed with an eerie silence. Even I, their only child, conceived so late in life, lived far away in the Himalayas, engrossed in my own life. No one seemed to need her any more. I wish I had been a little more patient and a little kinder to her. I wish I had told her how much I loved and admired her. I would have given anything to undo so many things. Regrettably, cochlear implants or the science of stem cell research and the incredible hope the sheer signage of regenerative medicine conjures up did not happen in my Mum's lifetime. She lived and died handicapped. An extraordinary human trapped in a silent world, waiting for information to filter down as a handout. *How cruel is that?*

Orphaned

When I met my Mum for the last time while I was on holiday from Nepal, she told me that she had many stories to tell me the next time I came home. Sadly, there was no next time. She passed away on 1st July 1984, before I saw her again. Her prayer that she be taken without being a burden to anyone was answered when she died on a Sunday morning within two hours of admission to the Apollo ICU after complaining of chest pain. Vimala, their tenant of many years, now family on all counts, was by her side in the ambulance and in the ICU in Apollo Hospital when she passed. When they brought her home and laid her to rest on her bed, family and friends poured in to say goodbye. Rekha and Anish were boarders at the Mount Hermon school in Darjeeling when Rev. Johnston, the principal, gently broke the news to them. Their beloved grandmother *Ammachy* who had looked after them as babies and during their school holidays, had passed away.

Posted in Kathmandu, Sam and I were the last to arrive. I remember walking into the room and stopping short in my tracks. My Mum had turned into a stranger in death. She was dressed in her wedding sari and looked completely at peace, but she was the colour of ebony. Refrigerated coffins had not reached Madras, and since my Dad would never have allowed her to be kept in a mortuary, the only option was to have her embalmed. Unfortunately, the morticians accepted her body only on Monday morning, twenty-four hours after her death, when rigor mortis had set in causing the lead oxide from the embalming fluid to leak into her tissues and discolour her skin.

I remember looking down at her lying in the coffin and thinking to myself, *this is not my Mum*! Losing a parent is a heart-breaking milestone no matter how old you are. It is an event that changes you forever – the end of an era, a status, and a lifetime of love. Life is never the same, ever again. *I knew that with my Mum gone, my life would never ever be the same again.*

Losing someone we take for granted is a hard pill to swallow. I would have done anything, *anything at all*, to have just five minutes alone with her. Five minutes to tell her how much I loved her and how sorry I was not to have understood her better. How sorry I was for all the times I was impatient, cross, and irritated because she could not hear or understand. How sorry I was that I took her for granted. How sorry I was not to have been kinder to her.

How I wish I had looked after her better. In all her relationships, she was the one who always did the caring and the looking after. Entitled, we just took her caring ways for granted. As I looked down at her lying still and immobile in the coffin, I knew that I would never be able to tell her all that I should have said when she was alive. Regret washed all over me in unrelenting waves as I realised that it was all over. My Mum had gone, and my life would never ever be the same again. I cannot even begin to explain the forlorn feeling that engulfed me as I crossed over a point of no return, numb and utterly alone.

Uncle VM Thomas buried my Mum, while my Dad watched silently as a grief-stricken spectator. I have never seen a man look more lost than he did when we turned to leave the cemetery. Death had finally separated them. She had left him months before their golden wedding anniversary, a milestone that incidentally coincided with him reaching fifty years as an ordained priest. He looked bereft and utterly devastated in a house full of relatives and friends. My Mum and Dad had not been apart for long spells since they were reunited after the war except for my Dad's sabbatical in Oxford at the Cuddeston College. The entries in the diary that my Dad kept over the weeks that followed were extremely raw and painful as he grieved privately for the loving companion who had stood beside him for so many years.

After my Mum passed away, I stayed with my Dad for two months to settle him into a life without my Mum. It was only after she left that I realised how hard she worked for the rest of us. She cooked every meal that came to the table. She never sat down until she had served us all. She never ate before making sure that our plates were full. She knew everyone's favourite preference and combination in food. She would move everything off the centre of the table so that she could see our plates and top up something that we had finished. How did we take her so much for granted?

The food that came to the table was a constant reminder

that my Mum had gone. Nothing tasted like her food though Bhaji, our Nepali man Friday, tried his best to replicate the recipes she had taught him. One day, my Dad and I decided to try making one of my Mum's signature dishes, the *meen patichathu*. We found the recipe that combined fish, grated coconut, and kokum in one of my Mum's Kerala cookbooks.

My Dad read out the recipe and I followed it word for word. Or so we thought. When it came to the table, it did not have the *chonna*, the pizazz, that we remembered from my Mum's dish. Going back to the recipe to see what had gone wrong, we laughed when we realised that my Dad had not turned the page and we had missed a few vital steps at the end, including the tempering of the dish with mustard, dry chillies, and onions. My Mum would have thrown up her hands in mock despair and said, *This Iyah is hopeless!*

After my Mum left, my Dad lost the will to live.

I was in London doing my dermatology training at St John's when I received his last blue aerogramme. He said that he was very tired and was waiting to go home. He always referred to heaven as home. *Be brave*, he wrote in his tidy handwriting with tiny letters that had never matched his persona or his frame. *Face life and all the challenges ahead, Susie, you will never be alone. God is with you. He will never leave your side,* he wrote, almost as if he was saying goodbye across the miles. A few days later, my cousin Leela called from Madras to say that my Dad had been admitted to the intensive care unit at Balaji Hospital down the road, in Guindy. The flights were going full, but the Air India staff went out of their way to be kind and helpful as they upgraded us to business class. We never knew how the hours passed as we sat strapped in our seats, fearful of what awaited us in Madras.

I think my Dad had a premonition. Before leaving for the

hospital, he crossed the road to the Bank of Baroda to sign some papers. He told them that I was on my way home and requested them to kindly help me when I arrived as I was not very good with money, banking, or accounts. He may even have remembered our hilarious sessions with his red hard-back copy of *Wren and Martin's English Grammar & Composition* when he tried so hard to teach me the correct way of writing official letters when I was growing up. He would want me to sign off as *yours faithfully* to the bank manager and I would flatly refuse saying that I would not be faithful to some strange old bank manager!

Bidding the Lhasa Apsos Tiny and Pappoo an emotional farewell, he handed Bhaji the house keys and said *Give it to Susie when she comes*. Vimala and Milner, their tenants upstairs, very kindly took my Dad to the hospital, where he walked in nursing a silent heart attack as diabetics are known to do. Sam and I reached Balaji Hospital two days before my Dad passed away. His eyes filled with relief when he saw me walk through the door as if he was waiting for me to come home. He struggled to speak, but he could not. He signalled for a pen, but it kept slipping from his hand as he tried repeatedly to write something. Exhausted, he eventually gave up and just lay there looking up at me with tears in his eyes. It broke my heart to see him like that.

Regret, remorse, and guilt chased each other down my cheeks as I looked down at him lying on the hospital bed. I could not believe that my Dad, the pivot of my life, was leaving me. I had just lost my Mum, and now my Dad too? Incredulously, I watched him slip away from me, leaving me behind utterly helpless, clinging on to his limp hand. I could not imagine a world without my Dad. The gentle giant who had always encouraged me to reach heights I never knew existed or thought I could scale. The kindest man I have ever known. The one who loved me unconditionally and whose eyes always lit up when I entered the room.

They put him on life support, for which they had to do a tracheostomy. I watched in mute horror as they chipped away at my Dad's eighty-year-old, calcified trachea. Every neuron in my brain silently screamed, *Stop*, while every painful beat of my heart clung to the slimmest hope of a miracle to help him survive and let me take him home. I was much younger and I did not understand terminal care then as I do today. *Why did I not make them stop? Did he need all that discomfort and pain at that point of his life? It would have been so much kinder to have let him go peacefully. Did I not see that there was not much more that they could have done? Did my grief as a daughter cloud my judgment as a doctor?* I now know that many of the futile end-of-life interventions carried out in an ICU are more for the family who watch helplessly and for the system, than for the patient. I now know better. If I knew then what I know now, I would have let him go quietly and peacefully. I would not be haunted by vivid visuals of him struggling during the tracheostomy. Sam was by his bedside when my Dad passed away on 10th March 1986. It was a Monday, at 7:30 in the evening, twenty lonely months after my Mum.

And just like that, my Dad slipped away quietly to a place I could not follow, leaving me behind. A place of no return as I clung desperately to my faith in a Risen Saviour and the assurance of a glorious reunion when I too would cross over. Never have I felt so alone as I did that night in a house overflowing with strangers, friends, and family. So very alone. Not lonely. Just alone.

The morticians embalmed him at home. They dressed him in his cassock and canon's cape and placed him in an open coffin in his study, the prayer room. His sanctum sanctorum, the room with an altar and a silver cross, where he celebrated the Holy Eucharist every day. As the embalming was done at home without any delay, he did not have any pigmentary changes and looked as if he were asleep. *Kochuttychaen* had arrived from Kerala to say goodbye to his beloved *Baboo Achen*, who had, together with his sister *Pengal*, looked after him all the years he worked in Singapore. His wife, *Achamma kochamma*, had passed away on 7th March in Kerala. Pushing aside his grief, he had come in an unreserved compartment on a crowded train from Kerala, standing all the way, the day after he buried his wife, to be with my Dad. He led the singing at the wake, lending his powerful baritone to every song without a break. Midway through the wake someone noticed that something was odd. My Dad looked different. No one could figure out what it was until someone realised that he was missing his glasses as he lay in the coffin. We scuttled around for them, searching high and low, but could not find them. Someone even went back to the hospital to look for them there, but they were nowhere to be found. No one found the glasses because they were perched on *Kochuttychaen's* nose. Well into the twentieth hymn or so, *Kochuttychaen* took off the glasses he was wearing and sheepishly announced that they could be my Dad's glasses. Distracted by all that was happening around him, he had picked up a pair of glasses lying on the piano to start the singing.

My Dad's wake lasted three nights as family and friends, including congregation members from Christ Church Singapore, flew in from all over the world to say goodbye. When my Mum and Dad had moved to Madras, we were working in Nepal and came home only on brief holidays. I had no idea that he had become such an integral part of the St Thomas Mount community in such a short time. I was astonished to see the house full and overflowing with the crowds that came to keep vigil, sing hymns, and pray continuously while waiting to attend his funeral. Bhaji ran the kitchen like a well-oiled machine, serving coffee and tea at regular intervals to the visitors while preparing the standard funeral fare of *kanji*, *pyaru*, and *chammandi*—hot rice porridge, green gram, and green mango chutney—for those who shared the family meals. Like other big families scattered across the globe who get to meet only at weddings and funerals, mealtimes during the wake are filled with fond reminiscences and family anecdotes laced with peals of laughter and tears.

A woman who did not leave my Dad's side the entire time had this story for me. She said that her husband had died one morning when the local pastor was away. Since all their near and dear ones lived close by there was no need to wait, and so she requested my Dad to conduct the funeral service the same afternoon.

My Dad, the *stepney* priest, agreed willingly. When the hearse arrived at the cemetery later that afternoon, the sun was shining. Halfway through the funeral service, the sky darkened without any warning, and soon, it started pouring. Everyone ran for cover except for my Dad, the corpse-in-the-casket, and his widow. The muddy grave slowly started filling up with rainwater. The coffin dislodged itself and started shifting, threatening to float up and out of the grave. Undeterred, my Dad finished all five pages of the funeral service under an umbrella, shielding the prayer book, not missing a comma or semicolon. There were no shortcuts in my Dad's *Book of Common Prayer*. Every single line was read out completely and with reverence. The lady said that she would never forget his dedication for as long as she lived, grateful that my Dad did not abandon the service midway. She was sure that anyone else would have stopped and continued only after the rains ceased.

Absolute strangers comforted me with kind words and anecdotes that spoke volumes about my Dad's support to them emotionally and financially. My Dad had one principle in life. If anyone ever came to him for a loan, he would never refuse. He would give them something so that they did not leave disappointed. What he gave, he never expected back. Many never returned it anyway, but it did discourage them from coming back and asking for more. I suspect that most of the time, he never told my Mum anything about these accounts. She would have rolled her eyes, thrown up her hands and said, *This Iyah is hopeless!*

My Uncle John Pothen—*Kunjootychaen*, sibling no. 18, my Dad's protégé—flew in from London to say goodbye to his mentor. My Dad had travelled to England shortly after my Mum passed away and watched with pride his youngest brother-in-law, a mere lad of ten, when they first met in Ettiyapuram decades ago, installed as a prebendary of St Paul's Cathedral in London.

My Dad was taken to the St Thomas Garrison Church on his way to the cemetery for a final visit to the church he loved. Intoning the final blessing, *Go forth in peace, thou faithful priest*, *Kunjootychaen* bade farewell to his beloved *Baboo Achen*. Uncle VM Thomas conducted the burial at the St Thomas Cemetery and wept throughout the entire service as he laid his friend to rest. For many years, they had met every Wednesday to celebrate the Holy Eucharist in my Dad's study and to have breakfast together after the service, a ritual they both enjoyed as retired priests. When he bid my Dad goodbye, he knew that he had lost a dear friend.

When my Mum died, there definitely was an outpouring of grief when the siblings and their families said goodbye to their *Pengal*. When my Dad died, the outpouring of grief was different. It was steeped in respect and gratitude as they said goodbye to the singularly unselfish man who had shared their *Pengal* with them after marriage and helped her look after the *Cadavanaltharayil* family. They mourned the passing of the young priest they had adopted nearly fifty years ago on a Sunday after church in Ettiyapuram, in South India. With his passing they lost a father figure, their beloved *Baboo Achen*.

Bhaji

Bhaji, our Nepali Man Friday, had relocated to the unfamiliar plains of Tamil Nadu to look after my Mum and Dad when they retired to Madras. He spoke no Malay, Tamil, or Malayalam, and my Mum and Dad spoke no Hindi or Nepali. They got by for many years with a brand of sign language they punctuated with audio-visuals and MMENT, a ludicrous mix of Malayalam, Malay, English, Nepali, and Tamil. Once when I pointed out that Bhaji didn't understand their mix of MMENT, my Mum, merely dismissed it with an impatient, *Hrmmmph. He should have learned it by now!* My Dad who had learned only a smattering of Malay words in all his thirty-three years in Singapore would tell him *Tengoh Bhaji* when at a loss for words, be it a directive, a question, or anything else. Dear faithful Bhaji stayed with my parents to the end. When my Dad passed, I had to close an empty house to return to London to continue my dermatology training at St John's. A tired Bhaji, who had chosen the sultry heat of Madras over the cool Himalayas, had to reluctantly admit that it was time to hang up his apron. He left, and we never saw him again. It was the end of an era, a lifetime of loyal devotion. He left as he came, silently and unobtrusively, taking our hearts full of love for him with him. Dear, dear Bhaji.

So many years

Though it has been many years since my Mum and Dad left me, I still miss them in the big things and the small. With every passing day, I have learned to live without them, but I have never forgotten their brand of tough love that has equipped me for life. I am an OCEP: an only child of elderly parents. A miraculous flash-in-the-pan when my Mum was an elderly primigravida at forty-six. I grew up blessed, loved, and cherished by two wonderful caring people I am proud to call my parents, my Mum and my Dad.

> Those we truly love never really die
> They live on in the love we shared
> The memories we treasure
> And in the assurance that we will meet again
> At His side when there will be
> No more tears and no more goodbyes

PART 4

St Margaret's | Stella Maris | CMC: Christian Medical College, Vellore | St John's Institute of Dermatology, London

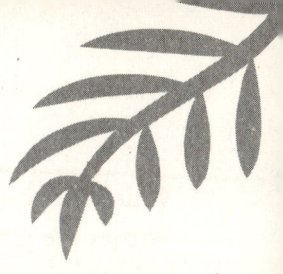

St Margaret's School

I was seven when I joined St Margaret's School, the oldest girls' school in the Far East. Founded in 1842 by Maria Dyer of the London Missionary Society, it grew from a boarding school that rescued abandoned Chinese girls, the *mui tsai*s from the streets, to become one of the finest girls' schools in Singapore, an Anglican government-aided school grounded firmly in Christian principles with its primary section on Sophia Road and the secondary on Farrer Road.

Most of us entered St Margaret's in the primary section and moved up en masse as a class. The primary school, spread out on a green hill near the *Istana* with Miss Norah Inge as the principal, is a dim but precious memory I treasure of my formative years until we moved to the secondary school in 1960. Our class of thirty was as cosmopolitan as indeed Singapore was. We celebrated our diversity by sharing our festivals. The Chinese shared the Mooncake Festival and Chinese New Year; the Christians, Christmas and Easter; the Muslims, Hari Raya Puasa and Haji; the Hindus, Diwali and Thaipusam, while our Jewish classmates shared Passover and Hanukah.

The school uniform was a green-and-white ensemble with white canvas shoes, calf-length white socks, and a green-and-white badge that stood for charity, patience, and devotion, virtues the school tried hard to impart to its students. Under our school uniform, at all times and in all places, we wore green bloomers. For those who have never met a pair of bloomers before, it is a bifurcated, baggy short knickerbocker elasticated at the waist and thigh. When we had PT or played netball, we merely stepped out of our skirts to run around the field in our green bloomers and white shirts, looking like a cross between an adolescent suffragist and a Tudor king, old-fashioned perhaps but superbly functional. If you were lying in the middle of the road after an accident, there would be nothing to fear as the bloomers covered everything.

Miss Isabel Lau

Our English teacher, Miss Isabel Lau, a diminutive cheongsam-clad lady, was a strict disciplinarian. Her mantra *There is always a better way* never allowed us to stagnate. When she made comprehension and précis a daily way of life, we realised that we would be handicapped if we did not have a vocabulary to help us shrink content without losing context.

Effortlessly, Miss Lau motivated us to build a personal lexicon by making us learn and use one new word a day. Failure to do so would land us squarely in her detention classes, a fate none of us enjoyed! Her commitment to her class was legendary. She had a Pygmalion effect on us that spurred us on, willing us to do well. *I will not accept less from you because I know you can do better,* she would say. We really had no choice, we just had to do better.

Mrs Phyllis Chin

Mrs Chin taught English Literature and Composition and we loved her. The prettiest teacher in the school in her floral, knee-length cheongsams, Mrs Chin never needed to raise her voice or lose her temper to get our attention; she had us wrapped around her little finger right from the start. The topics she handed out for composition were as varied as they were unusual and fired our imagination and creativity.

I loved Mrs Chin's composition classes. Though she never ever gave me more than 6 ½ on 10, seeing the quiet appreciation in her kind eyes when she returned our essays, I used to stretch in my socks, grow a few inches taller, and try harder. Mrs Chin was an intuitive teacher who nurtured us gently with love.

On our last day at school, she asked us if we understood the word *talent*. She listened to the thirty answers that tumbled out and smiled as she explained talent to a bunch of schoolgirls who were poised to take on the world.

> *It is a gift from God. Each one of you has a special 'something' that you will excel in. It will come naturally to you. You will never need to do a course or pass an exam for it. Identify your talents, girls; they will define you. Hone them. Share them. Enjoy them!* she said. *Remember, what you are, is God's gift to you, what you become is your gift to God.*

Every child should have a Mrs Chin in their life, a teacher who brings out the best in them.

Mrs Sushila Appadurai Cherian

When Sushila Appadurai, a stunning beauty and a concert pianist who excelled in sports as well, came to teach us English Literature, she had just been crowned *Deepavali Queen* at the Singapore University. St Margaret's had never had a beauty queen for a teacher and the excitement was palpable. She did *Hiawatha* with us and we christened her *Minnie-ha-ha, Laughing Waters,* hanging on her every word as we crowded around her desk. Actually, she did more than English Literature with us - she taught us social graces. Why she even taught us to sit like ladies in class with our legs together!

We were bereft when Sushila left for India to marry an officer in the Indian Navy, Dr Jickoo Cherian, the son of the governor of Maharashtra, Dr PV Cherian. A few years later, when Georgina, a classmate from St Margaret's and I were doing our pre-University in Stella Maris in Madras, we spent an afternoon with Sushila and Jickoo. They spun us around Madras in their red sports car with the hood down before they drove us to the Gymkhana Club for lunch. Georgina and I had never been to a club in our lives. We gawked and tripped as liveried men in colourful headgear saluted us and opened doors for us. Seated in the dining hall, in awe, we copied Sushila work her way through her cutlery across the table as we had never seen so many forks, knives or spoons next to our plates before and had no idea where to start. Bedazzled with our first brush with high society and high living, Georgina and I decided that when we finished college we were going to find ourselves men in uniforms like Jickoo to marry. Georgina did just that when she married Matt, a dashing young officer in the Indian Army!

Domestic science

St Margaret's equipped us with life skills to survive wherever we were planted. *No matter where your career takes you or does not take you, remember that you are homemakers.* They were right, and all that we learnt in the domestic science classes and the sewing classes came to my rescue in all the isolated places we worked in. Well, maybe not the sewing classes as I really did not enjoy the needle and thread. Perhaps if my Mum had been interested in needlework, I might have done better in my sewing classes.

My interest in cooking definitely stemmed from the attention my Mum paid to my domestic science classes. When I reached home after a domestic science period, which was usually the last one for the day, I would find my Mum waiting to inspect the dish I had prepared in class as she listened intently to a blow-by-blow account of Miss Sim Gai Kok's lesson. She would copy out the recipe from my workbook into her lined notebook, her *Recipe Book*, and make me practise what I had done in class at home so that she could learn it too. I think she was more interested in my domestic science recipe worksheets than she ever was in my report card. When Sam and I were posted to the Himalayan Kingdoms of Nepal and Bhutan, thanks to Miss Sim's domestic science classes, I was able to bake fresh bread and pastries in a temperamental Aga stove, without a timer and thermostat.

Mrs Martha Holloway

When we moved to Farrer Road in 1960, Mrs Holloway was the Principal of St Margaret's Secondary School, who had a heart of gold that she hid under a tough exterior. She was the one who sent us into the world after we finished our Senior Cambridge exams in 1962. The afternoon that I went in to pick up my results, I spent close to an hour in her room, seated across the desk from her. *Well done, Anne,* she said. She always called me Anne, the first of my many names. *You have done very well, and I am very proud of you;* she smiled one of her rare smiles of approval as she scanned my results. *What are you going to do now, Anne?*

I could not believe my ears. Here was someone wanting to know what I wanted to do. At home, I was always told what to do. My Mum wanted me to become a doctor. Aptitude and career counselling never existed in her vocabulary, neither in English nor in Malayalam. I had to do medicine, and that was it. My Dad never opposed her once her mind was set as he would have ended up talking to a wall.

Why can't I be a lawyer? I whined when I finished reading the Perry Mason series. The thought of brushing aside the defence's evidence as *irrelevant, immaterial, and inconsequential* was quite intoxicating.

Lawyers have to tell lies to save their clients, Susie, they both said in a tired voice. *You know how you get caught every time you lie,* they said, exchanging knowing looks. *If you have to lie to save people, they will all swing.*

Why can't I do journalism? I asked, whining afresh on a new pitch. *I may end up being rich and famous,* I said, brightening at the thought of bookstores displaying my books and my pen running dry from signing autographs.

You must have a steady income, they said in a tired voice that really translated into: *After our time, what will happen to you?* They were great drama queens when they set their minds to emotional blackmail. *You must be independent,* they said emphatically. And that was that.

Career options for girls in the early 1960s were fairly limited as most girls grew up sheltered under a sky where only men flew aeroplanes. *Go be a doctor, go be a teacher, go be a nurse,* the Indian diaspora told their daughters. We were expected to make career choices wearing gender as a restrictive collar around our necks. My Mum's monotone had only one refrain. *Go be a doctor... Go be a doctor... Go be a doctor... Go!* With this scenario at home, I looked up hopefully when Mrs Holloway asked me what I wanted to do.

Perhaps I could persuade Mrs Holloway to talk to my Mum and Dad, I thought. *Surely they will never be able to say no to her.* I could not imagine anyone refusing Mrs Holloway, and it certainly would not hurt to have her in my corner. I sat up and presented my opening remarks. I told her that my Mum and Dad wanted me to do medicine, whereas I wanted to be a lawyer. I told her about my courtroom fantasies, à la Perry Mason style, where I saw myself in a black coat dismissing evidence as *irrelevant, immaterial, and inconsequential*. She picked up the phone and tried talking my Mum and Dad out of medicine as an option for me. It did not make a dent. What was worse, she did a mental flip and ended up on their side. She even told me that she wished she had done medicine!

It's a noble profession, Anne, she pronounced. *You will be better off in the white coat. Forget the black,* she said. Utterly defeated, I left her room. I had played my last stallion, lost the battle, and was trundled off to the pre-med class in St Andrew's School, and the rest is history.

I lost touch with Mrs Holloway until I visited her in the hospital many years later. I looked down at her through the tears in my eyes. This was not the iron lady who had struck terror into my very soul during all our escapades in school. *What happened here?* I asked myself as I leaned forward to hear what she was saying. *How are you doing, Anne? Enjoying the white coat?* she asked me in a faint whisper.

Fine, I gulped, amazed that she remembered our last meeting. She reached out and took my hand. *Anne, I am so happy that you did medicine,* she said. *Study hard and help people like me,* she smiled. *Now come and kiss me goodbye and leave,* she said as she dismissed me. She could have been in her office behind her desk at that moment, not lying helplessly on her back in a hospital bed. *Kiss Mrs Holloway?* I swallowed incredulously. *That would be like kissing God!* I bent down fearfully and kissed her goodbye. I was leaving a wonderful human being who had indelibly shaped my life. Someone I will never ever forget.

Think outside the box

St Margaret's did not confine our education to the pages of our book. We were taught to think outside the box and to improvise. We were penalised if we regurgitated pages of rote learning, and we actually lost marks if our answers looked even remotely like the text in our books. Private tuitions at home implied that you were a mutt and were not encouraged. We were expected to work on our own with help from our teachers in class. St Margaret's gave me a distinct advantage and a head start in all the colleges and courses I attended later. And I am truly grateful.

When I look back, I see a sea of faces: dedicated teachers who moulded us through all our young and unlovable years. Teachers who never gave up on us, who cared enough to see beyond us, into our future. I am grateful, deeply, deeply grateful to every single one of them.

A stranger rewrites my destiny

Six months into my pre-med classes in St Andrews School, my life took a sudden and unexpected turn, thanks to the advice of a visitor who was passing through Singapore. The visitor worked with a missionary group in India, and by the end of his stay, he had convinced my Mum and Dad that I would be better off doing a Pre-University Course (PUC) in India. This would prepare me for the entrance exams to one of the many medical colleges in India. No one bothered to ask me what I wanted to do or where I wanted to study. On his return to India, the missionary gentleman got me admitted to the PUC in Stella Maris College and appeared at Madras Port as my local guardian when I got off the ship. An absolute stranger had changed the whole course of my destiny. And I let it happen as an out-of-body experience.

One evening, a green tin trunk measuring 4'×2'×2' with Anne Baboo painted on the lid in white appeared in the parsonage sitting room. With an unusual flurry of shopping and packing, I suddenly found that I had a new wardrobe, new shoes, and new toiletries that went into a pretty, new toilette bag. New everything. If I had asked for the moon, my Mum and Dad would have flown up to pluck it out of the sky and thrown in a few stars too. As the trunk filled, my Mum and Dad debated whether my genealogy and vital statistics should be painted on the trunk. To my enormous relief, just the name won. My green trunk and I were put on the ship, *SS Rajulah*, with my friend Mercy Mathews and all the other students bound for further studies in India.

When I left home in the summer of 1963, I saw my Dad cry for the first time in my life. In my excitement, I never noticed how sad they were when the ship pulled away from the harbour. I skipped up the undulating gangplank with all the other students bound for India, and sailed away from the wharf, the island, the family, and the parsonage blissfully unaware that my life would never be the same ever again.

Stella Maris, Madras

After the admission formalities, the green trunk and I were safely ensconced in a room at the Lady's Hostel with my Malaysian roommates, Mary Rajah, Susie Samuel, and Lily Harris. Away from home for the first time, we bonded instantly as buddies in a healthy mix of mischief and sobriety. Sister Carla Rosa, the Principal of Stella Maris College, a beautiful nun from Europe, was an excellent pianist. When she played the national anthem, she would turn to us and call out in her lilting Italian accent, *Girls, we will now sing the Janaganamana*. Only when she started the music would we recognise the national anthem. She did not like boys. Nor did she like brothers visiting their sisters in the hostel. She had a very simple and logical explanation for a rule she never broke. *Your brother is not her brother,* she would say, pointing randomly at the crowd. *Or hers. Or hers.* Brothers, as far as she was concerned, were potentially dangerous, and cousins with a Y chromosome simply did not exist.

We were allowed to go out on Saturday afternoons until 6 pm. Our favourite haunts were the Buhari Hotel and the Southern Chinese restaurant on Mount Road. The prices were affordable, the helpings generous, and most importantly, it was not hostel food that we cribbed about incessantly. If we returned late to the hostel, we were gated. The watchman at the gate could not be bribed or bullied as one of the nuns stood beside him, armed with pencil and notebook, gleefully jotting down the names of late-comers.

On Sundays, the protestant students were allowed to attend the morning service at St George's Cathedral down the road. The visits to the cathedral were not fuelled by any religious fervour. We went only because it was an extra outing and an opportunity to eat at the drive-in Woodlands opposite the cathedral, where all the rich and famous, film stars included, would hang out.

PU-7

Our regular day started with study time, breakfast, and assembly, after which we were let loose to attend our classes. Most of us, the students from Singapore and Malaya, in the PU-7 class wore dresses that fell to our knees. Filing out after assembly, we were asked to step aside if our hemline was even a hairbreadth above our knee. We had to rip the seam and let the fabric hang modestly over our knees. Knees were not meant to be seen; knees were mere orthopaedic appliances made by God to connect the thigh to the leg; knees would come to ruin if they were left uncovered.

We were introduced to French as our second language for the exams. Even the girls who had studied Tamil in Malaysia took French as their second language. This was a smart move as the French we did was so basic we even surprised ourselves by scoring distinctions in the exams that pushed our grades up.

1963 revisited

Fifty-seven years later, in 2020, I heard a voice from the past. Lilly Harris found my profile on Facebook and sent me a message. Delighted, we decided to trace as many of *the old gang* as we could. Lilly promptly set up a WhatsApp group and named it *Stella Maris 1963* with a black-and-white photograph from her album and circulated it on social media. Before we knew it, we had found many more, including our roommates Susie and Mary, as well as Georgina, Mercy, Lakshmi, Raji, Subba, and Indira, for an emotional cyber reunion. Soon sepia photographs of young teenagers came cascading in as everyone posted old memories and long-forgotten anecdotes, a sharp contrast to the more recent colour pictures of unrecognisable septuagenarians with their pets, gardens, husbands, kids, and grandkids. God, in His infinite mercy, had sent us another treasured distraction to cushion our sunset years. We hold on to these renewed ties with grateful hearts as the easy friendships of our youth resurfaced.

The Christian Medical College entrance exams

After our PUC exams, a bunch of us from Stella Maris wrote the entrance exams for CMC Vellore, at the breezy Madras University building, on Marina beach. When we arrived, the place was packed and overflowing with hopeful aspirants and anxious parents who hovered over their wards, plying them with food, drink, and last-minute advice. Huddled together on the grounds outside, we felt like orphans with no one to fuss over us. Shrugging aside the forlorn feeling, we convinced ourselves that the entrance exam was no big deal. It was just another hurdle to get over. Clueless about what awaited us, we nonchalantly took our places in the hall.

It was a written paper with multiple-choice questions, including mental ability tests. Several fascinating pages of problem-solving and mental ability followed the sections on science and general knowledge. Though we enjoyed the mental floss, we had no way of assessing how we had done or if we would make it to CMC. Nor did we know that thousands of students were writing these tests in centres all over India at the same time. We had no clue that only a hundred and twenty would be called for a three-day interview in CMC Vellore when sixty successful candidates, thirty-five boys and twenty-five girls, would be selected to join the first year MBBS class. What we did not know did not worry us as we headed towards the Marina Buhari's to stuff our faces singing while the juke box in the restaurant played Doris Day's *Que sera sera*.

My Mum and Dad arrived from Singapore when I finished my PUC exams. Packed and ready, I was raring to start my holiday with my *Annammal Paatti* and my cousins in Kodukulanji. My Mum and Dad ran around like a pair of headless chickens all summer, getting all my certificates in order for admission to a medical college. I just signed the admission forms whenever and wherever they asked me to sign. It was clear that they were not going back to Singapore until they had me admitted into a medical college somewhere in India. I was accepted by Madras Medical College, where my Mum had done her shortened MBBS course. Though my Mum and Dad were pleased and relieved, I knew that they were hoping that I would be admitted to CMC, where my Mum had done her LMP thirty-nine years earlier.

Aunt Ida

My Mum was deeply influenced by the life and work of Dr Ida Sophie Scudder, the founder of CMC Vellore. Ida Scudder, a young American girl, had a life-changing experience while visiting her parents who were working as missionaries in South India. During her stay in Dindivanam, a village south of Vellore, the family was woken up in the middle of the night by a desperate and poignant cry for help, a cry that changed Ida Scudder's life and the lives of many young people through the ages.

In the span of a single night, three young men came desperately seeking help late for their wives in labour and left disappointed when they heard that the doctor was not a woman. The conservative villagers wanted a lady doctor to attend to their women in labour. Ida was devastated. Three young girls died in childbirth for want of a lady doctor, and they took their babies with them. Troubled by the events of that fateful night, Ida Scudder turned her back on love and marriage and joined Cornell University's medical school in the US. She decided she would return to India as a doctor to help those in need, especially the women and children who were kept in pitiable conditions in their homes. When she completed her medical training, she returned to Vellore and set up a one-bed mission station in 1900 and a medical school for women in 1918. Cradled in prayer, this grew into a two thousand–bed multi-speciality hospital and a coed medical college of international repute: the Christian Medical College Vellore.

My Mum was enrolled for the LMP course in 1925. Thus,

she left hearth and home, the siblings, and all things familiar to go on a journey that changed the entire course of her life. She was one of the earlier ones taught by Dr Ida Scudder, Aunt Ida, as she was known to her doting students.

My Mum and Dad were taking no chances when it came to my admission to CMC. They had come armed with a sponsorship from the SPG Mission in Singapore as my Dad was serving as the *Pathriyar* of the Tamil congregation of Christ Church and as a Canon of the St Andrew's Cathedral, Diocese of Singapore. Every year, 75 per cent of the students admitted to CMC are sponsored by churches or missions that support the college. In return for the education, the sponsored students are required to sign a service bond and work for a stipulated time in the hospitals run by the missions. If I got into CMC Vellore sponsored by the SPG in Singapore, I was expected to return to Singapore and work at St Andrew's Hospital, the hospital associated with the SPG Mission.

Somewhere in the middle of my glorious holiday with my Kodukulanji cousins, I received a postcard inviting me to attend the selection interview at CMC. I had crossed the first hurdle.

The CMC admission interviews

Unfortunately, the heat and the excitement leading up to my CMC selection interview were too much for my Mum, who fell ill. Leaving her behind in Kodukulanji, my Dad and I travelled to Katpadi, the railway station closest to Vellore. My first glimpse of the college took my breath away. Massive granite buildings surrounded by hills nestled in a green oasis with the chapel in the sunken garden as a picturesque backdrop of tranquillity and peace. It really seemed like a place set apart. Parents accompanying the interview candidates were asked to find hotels in town and return only after three days when the results would be announced. We were then assigned to senior students for accommodation in the hostels. Mary C George, one of my fifty-seven cousins who was a final year student, took me up to her room and settled me in. After lunch, I joined the others in the beautiful sunken garden, where we were split into groups of ten and given number tags to wear. Mine was ninety-eight. Our group observers, Dr Zareena Isaac and Mrs Abraham Verghese, as different as chalk and cheese, complemented each other seamlessly as they shepherded us through the selection. For three days, we moved like geese. We went everywhere with them, and we did everything with them. They each carried a file into which they entered mysterious notes as they looked us up and down mentally. Initially, this worried us enough to put us on our best behaviour, but eventually, we forgot that we were being watched or assessed and slipped into our usual boisterous selves.

Our group was a motley crew, a mismatch of young girls from all over India and overseas. We had only one thing in common: having come this far in the competition, we all wanted to get into CMC. The interviews lasted the whole day when we were given mental ability and IQ tests to solve. We were allotted tasks to complete individually and as a group, and graded by unknown parameters to assess our skills as individuals and as team players. The group observers quizzed us individually about our families, our religious beliefs, our dreams, and our aspirations. When we returned at night, the seniors would be waiting up for us, curious to know how we had done. Unfortunately, we had no clue as the entire selection process was completely new and an unfamiliar experience.

After three days, we were sent off on a picnic with the seniors while the selection committee fine-tuned the final list.

We were taken around to see the wonders of Vellore, which included a river with no water, a fort with no king, and a temple with no idol. We bounced around in the bus, singing all the bawdy songs that we had picked up effortlessly, pushing the uncertainty of the admissions to the ill-lit back burners of our young minds. *Are you coming to Vel-Vellore* was a popular ditty, translated and sung in Hindi, Tamil, Malayalam, Telegu, Kannada, and all the languages commonly spoken in India and in Malay and Chinese for the students from Singapore and Malaysia. *Are you coming to Vel-Vellore, Are you coming to Vel-Vellore? Tell me true, my darling, Are you coming to Vel-Vellore?*

When they took us to the mortuary, the unfamiliar smell of formalin stung our eyes. On one of the steel tables lay a silhouette covered with a white sheet from head to toe. We were told that he had just died and his body had been donated for dissection. Many of us had never seen a dead body before, and this was our first brush with mortality. We stood there frozen as we gazed in awe and respect, mesmerised by the sight, the smell, and the silence of death. Suddenly the silence was shattered when the silhouette leapt up, threw off the sheet with a blood-curdling yell, *Aaaauuuuaauuaaaa aaaaaaaaaaaah*, and jumped off the table. Petrified, we ran, shrieking in terror as the seniors watched with unbridled amusement. Every year this act scared the living daylights out of the interview candidates.

After lunch, we huddled in the sunken garden outside the college chapel as an unseen voice called out the final list of selected candidates over a microphone. The ones who had cleared the interview gravitated to one side of the divide, separating them from those who had not. Those on the waiting list were not entirely without hope, as a few on the final list inevitably discontinued or transferred, allowing the candidates on the waiting list to join later. Four of us—Joyce Ponnaiya,

Elizabeth Ninan, Florence Blandina, and I—were selected from the ten in our group.

Tears usually meant that you had not got in. My Dad was quite bewildered when he saw me sobbing uncontrollably. *Why are you crying?* he asked. *You're in. What's wrong with you? Are you not well?* he asked, looking extremely worried as I continued to sob inconsolably. All my friends from Stella Maris who had come for the interview with me were going back, leaving me behind. And suddenly, they did not seem very friendly either. The sunken garden emptied quickly as the seniors bundled us away into the hostel to rag us. My Dad left after a hurried goodbye, promising to be back in a few days with my Mum and my green trunk.

We were a privileged bunch, selected from a long list of applicants and enrolled in an exclusive, premier medical college. The feeling could be intoxicating if allowed to develop. We might even grow a few obnoxious horns that would need lopping off. Ragging would take care of the arrogance and cut us down to size.

Ragging

Ragging in the women's hostel was never physical. It was playful and verbal, with watchful seniors quick to rap the knuckles of the overenthusiastic younger seniors who may have crossed an invisible line. We had two options: either we played the sport or we sulked. If we pretended to enjoy ourselves, the seniors lost interest and left us alone. If we sulked, we cried out for more.

We were assigned fag mistresses, seniors who were supposed to keep an eye on us. Mine was Ari Kumari, a Malaysian in the final year. She would watch me from the corner of her eye to make sure that I was not bullied. When she thought I needed a break, she would summon me to her room and feed me snacks and goodies like sour cannas and biscuits from Malaysia. Handing me a giant stitching needle and some coloured wool, she would, in a stern voice say, *Stitch two hearts on my carpet by the time I return.* Closing the door, she would leave me with some peace and quiet. Her carpet was full of hearts stitched by other freshers from previous batches that she had rescued for short breaks. Dear Ari, my fag mistress with a heart of gold. Decades later, we met again when we moved to Madras, and she went back to looking after me. Whenever she returns from her holidays abroad, she sends me a bag of goodies, stuffed and overflowing. The bond between a fag mistress and a fresher is usually built to last a lifetime.

We looked ludicrous in the fancy dress they made us wear as they paraded us around the women's hostel with lipstick and eye make-up smeared all over our faces. Our hair, braided medusa-style, was tied up in mismatched colourful ribbons, making us look like kathakali dancers sporting Afro wigs. When they insisted that I sing a Malay song, I bleated out Aneke Gronloh's *Burong Kaka Tuah*, and they all chimed in, drowning the chorus *la croom, la croom, ooh la la* with *bathroom-bathroom-bathroom-ooh-la-la*.

Subbalakshmi, a senior, taught us the *Kumbakkonam* dance. She placed us in rows with our hands on our hips, grooving to the hippie-hippie shake and swinging from side to side as she sang *Kumbakkonam-Kumbakkonam- Kum-kum-kum*. It was so hard to keep a straight face when we all looked so silly, we would end up giggling and falling about. Shouts of *look sharp, wipe that smile* would have us straightening up and gyrating as a group again. The early morning mass drill in the quadrangle of the women's hostel, had us in rows facing the seniors running up and down blowing shrill whistles. We were ordered to clench our fists with our elbows at right angles and pull them back and forth in a rowing movement. This resulted in our chest pumping up and out as we chanted, *I must, I must increase my bust.*

At the end of three days, we were taken back to the sunken garden for the final ducking ceremony, the rite of passage to the women's hostel of CMC. Blindfolded, we were led by our fag mistresses to Maya Tampi, the general secretary of the women's hostel. Prising open our mouths, they poured in a revolting cocktail of aubergines, okra, and all things slimy, which they called *The Nectar of Toads*. Blindfolded, we protested and puked, half-swallowing and half-spitting the disgusting concoction. *Yew... Yuck... Phew!* We were then picked up, swung by our hands and feet, and flung unceremoniously into the lily pond bringing the ragging to an official end. A hot bath and several welcome hugs later, we sat down as honoured guests to a special dinner, where we were officially welcomed into the fraternity of the women's hostel.

Several things happened quite imperceptibly in those three remarkable days. After being put through the wringer of ragging, we had no delusions of grandeur. Nor did we have time to be homesick or mope. The seniors and the freshers interacted long and well enough to make friends across the years. And most importantly, faced with the common challenge of dodging the seniors, the freshers bonded to become a protective band that looked out for their batchmates.

Kiddies Korner

Normally, new students who cleared the interview lived in the women's hostel with their seniors. Only two batches, the girls of 1963 and 1964, lived with Miss Mary Poonnen, the warden of Kiddies Korner, the little house next to the Scudder Auditorium. Set apart and singled out, Ma Poonnen, as she was fondly called, safely out of earshot, and the fresher girls of the batch of 1964 were sitting ducks for the seniors. They resented the restrictions on ragging caused by the isolation of freshers in a separate building. However, nothing could keep the seniors from surprising us almost every day with their innovative pranks. Every time we got ducked with water balloons, Ma Poonnen was drenched emotionally. When they serenaded us, they leaned heavily against her pane, pun totally intended.

An excellent cook, Miss Poonnen would sound the gong at mealtimes. We would sit down to gourmet food in dainty helpings that merged with the designs on her bone china plates. Fine dining with exquisite dishes served with artistry did not impress us teenagers who were hungry all the time. Sundays were special, as Ma Poonnen took a break and sent us off to the women's hostel for Sunday lunch and dinner.

The chicken pieces would be served on round white plates set on the wooden tables. If we closed our eyes during the singing of grace at Sunday lunch, there was a strong possibility that the chicken piece, the leg or breast in front of us, would fly into someone else's plate and disappear forever. Goolu, my classmate and friend would stand in front of the chicken leg, and I would stand in front of the chicken breast and sing grace with our eyes wide open, shamelessly watching our chicken pieces with an unwavering gaze.

When the late-comers urged us to move along so that they could shuffle in, we pretended to be totally engrossed in singing the grace. We did not move or blink, and we never took our eyes off the plate in front of us. Sunday dinner was a head-and-neck chicken curry cooked with giblets, offal, and the bishop's nose. This delicious rustic recipe was served out of steel buckets held by curved handles that clanged noisily when set down, buckets that looked suspiciously like the ones in the labour room and the operation theatres. We did not care how it was served. It was chicken, and any whiff of the bird would do.

Miss Poonnen conducted prayers at 8 pm before our study time. We would spend hours choosing unfamiliar hymns and deliberately sing them off-key to wrong tunes just to mess up her carefully planned timetable. This could be distinctly awkward as the melody would sometimes end before the lyrics did, leaving extra words fraught with uncertainty, suspended in mid-air, with no tune to finish with. This would have us in splits and Ma Poonnen up in arms, shattering the religious thermostat she tried so hard to set, night after night. Over the months, the practical jokes at Kiddies Korner graduated from amateur to genius. Each one more brilliant than the last, was choreographed and executed with an incredible eye for detail. We never knew who or what would strike next as neither Miss Poonnen nor all the watchmen were a match for the innovative seniors. One night, there was utter confusion in the dorm. Roma, in her baby doll pyjamas, was jumping up and down on her bed screaming at the top of her voice, and a bunch of girls who crowded around her were screaming with her. Lying on the bed was a silhouette covered with her blanket. Miss Poonnen rushed up to the bed and pulled the blanket away in one fell swoop. There lying on Roma's bed was a fully articulated skeleton.

It's Mr Tee, screeched someone. *Look, it's Mr Tee!* Indeed it was *Mr Tee*, the loose-limbed skeleton that usually hung suspended from a stand at the entrance of the anatomy dissection hall. Every morning, he would greet everyone with his clicking jaw as they brushed past him into the anatomy hall. *Mr Tee* was lying on Roma's bed, and what was worse, he had one femur crossed nonchalantly over the other. Truth be told, he looked as if he was grinning impudently from ear to ear. He looked very comfortable, very cosy, and very much at home in Roma's bed. Miss Poonnen was livid. The expletives she belted out in English and Malayalam that night cannot be repeated. This was a major security lapse as there was no way that *Mr Tee* could have walked up the steps on his own. *Skeletons do not walk up two flights of stairs,* she hissed through gritted teeth. We knew that. We knew that he had been carried up to the dorm and deposited on Roma's bed, on Ma Poonnen's watch. Everyone knew who had done it, but no one squealed, and the pranks continued.

The pre-clinical years: First year

Our subjects in first year included physics, chemistry, biology, English, Tamil, biostatistics, Bible class, and *sorting out our class boys*. By the time we had finished with the boys in our batch, they could spell *EQUALITY* backwards and blindfolded. We were a class of *alpha dog* personalities with high IQs, a result of an experiment in the selection process that year which we discovered later, and everyone marched to their own drumbeat. We never agreed on anything and we could never complete a class meeting without someone walking off in a huff. The boys and girls never really jelled like the other batches did, earning us the title of *The Disintegrated Batch*. It took fifty years of being knocked around in the big bad world for us to appreciate each other. At our Golden Jubilee in 2016, forty-six survivors from the batch of sixty-four from all over the world met and flew into each other's arms, making tender enquiries about the health, wealth, and happiness of the other. Apparently, we got on better as mature adults than we did as teenagers. Sam and I were the elected class reps in our first year, and it is still a mystery how we ended up together and stayed together all these years.

The NCC, the Old Moustache, and the sad sacks

While Miss Poonnen struggled with moulding our character, the National Cadet Corps, the NCC, struggled with our two left feet and the flag. The day we joined the NCC, we stood in a single file on the arid cricket oval in Bagayam and signed up for a set of khaki uniforms, a beret, a belt, a buckle, socks, and a pair of heavy-duty leather boots. The pathetic khaki was an unflattering one-size-fits-all that reduced us into shapeless, sad sacks.

We marched merrily along in single file and on the double, week after week, month after month, completely unprepared for what lay ahead at the end of the first year. Just before the final exams, the Old Moustache barked out that we would have to return the khaki uniforms, washed, ironed, and accounted for with all the accessories the next day if we wanted to collect our hall tickets for the exams.

We were catatonic for the rest of the nightmare as soap and water had not met sock and uniform in weeks. *Where on earth would we find a dhobi to launder the uniforms in 24 hours? How can we wash off all that dirt in a single night?* We wondered in shock. *How would we explain this to our parents? That we were not allowed to do our first year exams because we had not laundered our NCC uniforms and returned them in perfect condition?* Good grief, we would all have gotten an earful from home!

That night, the good little kiddies sat up all night to do their NCC laundry and hang it out in the balcony to dry. One wicked little kiddie lied through her back teeth and said she would wash her khakis the next morning and slept blissfully while the good little kiddies slaved. The wicked little kiddie, who wishes to remain anonymous, had an outrageous plan in mind and never washed anything in the morning. She merely bunked Mr Kunder's English class at 3 pm the next day and ran all the way home to Kiddies Korner. Hurriedly, this wicked little kiddie randomly pinched two sets of clean uniforms from the khakis that hung over the balcony. Yawning gaps on the clothesline were quickly filled with smelly substitutes, several shades deeper than khaki. The wicked little kiddie then ran all the way to Old Moustache, returned the laundered khakis, socks, boots, buckle, and beret before hiding in the library pretending to study and returning to Kiddies Korner only when it was dark. The unsuspecting good little kiddies were confused when they returned to find unwashed smelly khakis interspersed between the clean ones they had left to dry. Good-natured angels that they were, they thought they had missed a few and washed out the dirty khakis, earning them business class tickets to heaven with no stops anywhere.

All's well that ends well, and between all of us, we managed to return all the uniforms to the officer, collect our hall tickets, write the exams, and pass with flying colours. This secret, closely guarded for over fifty years, has now been released with indemnity cover.

Friendships forged under duress survive time and distance, especially when everyone watches everyone's back. Bonding under these circumstances is totally devoid of pretence. These low maintenance friendships of our teens survived well into our septuagenarian years to span all the milestones of our lives. The girls of the 1964 batch who started out in Ma Poonnen's Kiddies Korner turned out to be an unforgettable star-studded cast of trailblazers in their own right. *Each one more stunning than the other!*

After our batch, Kiddies Korner was scrapped as the seniors protested against the fragmentation of the women's hostel and wanted everyone under one roof. I do not think any of us ladies of the 1964 batch would ever trade the memories we shared at

Kiddies Korner for anything in the world. I know I would not.

The pre-clinical years
We soon moved into the second year to do anatomy, physiology, and biochemistry. The Anatomy Hall, a grey building with a high compound wall at the end of the basketball court, was an enigma. I could never understand why dead bodies needed a high wall to guard them. Most of the bodies used for dissection came from the Central Jail in Vellore town, while others were unclaimed bodies from the hospital mortuary.

A dead body is a corpse. When the corpse is used for medical or scientific purposes, it becomes a cadaver. We learnt anatomy hands-on through the dissection of cadavers, fixed in formalin to preserve them. These cadavers, in part or whole, were stored in formalin-filled cement tanks with a customised metal lid that could be lifted upwards and rested against the wall when the tanks had to be opened. When cadavers were needed for dissection, the attenders would stand on a stool and fish them out using mean-looking iron hooks welded to the end of a wooden pole.

The cadavers were dismembered into different parts. When a tank was agitated, cadaver parts would float up in silence. Sometimes, a limb floated up. Occasionally, a head bobbed up and down looking at us with sightless eyes before it went back in. Initially, this rather bizarre display of grey human parts would unnerve us, and we used to look away, acutely uncomfortable.

After a while, we became so acclimatised to the cadavers, the smell of formalin, and dissection that we forgot they were human beings who had once walked this earth like us. We forgot that they belonged to families and may have been someone's parent, sibling, or child. Had they any inkling that the body they had bathed, washed, and clothed would be a learning tool in clumsy student hands? Did they ever think that they would contribute to the pursuit of knowledge in medical science? Were they watching from a distance as we dissected our way to a better understanding of the human body? Sometimes we wondered what they were like, these forlorn bodies that floated up periodically. Most times, they were just parts to be dissected: an upper limb, a lower limb, a head, a neck, a thorax, an abdomen, a pelvis, mere objects to learn on.

For many of us, this was our first vision of nudity. One of the girls in our batch, the eldest of five sisters, had never seen a naked man in her life. All these male parts lying around in gay abandon was too much for her. She was fine when she worked on the upper and lower limbs. She had no problem dissecting the head and neck. She sailed through the abdomen and the thorax. But when it came to the pelvis and the male reproductive organs, it was a different ball game. One morning, she sat down at the table totally unprepared, thinking that the part for dissection was a sagittal section of the face, cutting through the nose. When she heard that what lay before her was the male pelvis, and that was no nose, she shot out of her stool like a rocket leaving the launch pad. She sat with her back to the table during all the sessions on the male reproductive anatomy that followed, giggling hysterically. All this nudity, albeit grey and in formalin, impacted her young mind so much that she chose to specialise in anaesthesia so she could safely stay at the head end of the patient.

In our practical classes in physiology, we did experiments on pithed frogs. The pithed frog was a model used in experimental physiology to show that some vertebrates can survive and demonstrate purposive behaviour, even swim, without a brain. This explained human behaviour on so many different levels.

The cadavers in the Anatomy Hall did not freak me out as much as a pithed frog did, moving limbs that were pinned down even as it lay brainless on an experimental plate!

The clinical years

Soon we were clinical students, riding the blue bus to the hospital to see patients. We felt like real doctors in our pinned and pleated saris and white coats with our hair up. We walked through the wards with our new Littman stethoscopes slung nonchalantly around our necks, feeling supremely important. We shared learning with our seniors in the air-conditioned auditorium for the integrated classes when the senior faculty took us through normal anatomy and physiology, pathology, clinical presentation, diagnosis, differentials, treatment, and prognosis in disease, replete with live case presentations, another first for us.

We were rotated in batches through all the departments in the hospital. Dr Shanti Fenn's surgical clinics in the afternoons were resoundingly popular and usually packed to overflowing as his diagnostic and surgical skills were legendary. As a teacher, he explained the most complicated events in surgery in the simplest way possible, leaving indelible impressions. We could never make out what went on in his head as he always had an inscrutable expression. He would never interrupt the student who was presenting the case. He would listen dispassionately to the presentations as students tied themselves up in knots trying to impress him, absolutely in awe of the man.

Dr Fenn's clinics

One afternoon, we were assigned a new patient to work up for the surgical clinic. The patient, a young man, sheepishly pointed to his right middle finger and said, *I have an ulcer that goes from here to there.*

We grabbed his right hand and examined his middle finger. There was nothing there. We pulled his fingers apart and examined all his fingers to find nothing. When questioned if he had an ulcer anywhere else, he denied it vehemently. We gave him back his right hand and marched purposefully over to the other side of the bed. We then grabbed his left hand and examined all the fingers. Not a scratch on his left hand. Intrigued, we asked him again if he had anything, at which point he started getting annoyed and hastily retrieved both his hands and hid them behind his back. Puzzled, we went off for coffee, wondering if he had been assigned to us to hone our history-taking skills. None of us suspected that we had missed anything.

One of the girls in our batch, a shy pretty young thing, presented the curious case of the ulcer that travelled up and down on the right middle finger to Dr Fenn. Engrossed in the presentation, none of us noticed that the patient was becoming increasingly uncomfortable as the clinic wore on. In conclusion, the shy young thing triumphantly declared the patient as a case of a healed ulcer on the right middle finger. She thought she had done rather well and was beginning to glow with confidence as she finished and looked up at Dr Fenn. Without batting an eyelid, Dr Fenn turned to the patient and signalled with his right index finger. *Drop your pants*, he said, *Show them what you have.* And there, in all its glory, lay the mysterious ulcer that moved up and down along his right middle finger. We were mortified! The shy young thing, who is now a grown woman of the world and is no longer shy or young but still very pretty, blushes a deep shade of crimson when this story is recounted at every reunion.

Dr Frank Garlick's surgical board

Dr Frank Garlick, a deeply committed Australian surgeon, introduced us to the textbook *Bailey and Love's Short Practice of Surgery*. When he treated a patient, they were not just X, Y, or Z or bed number 1, 2, or 3. They were definitely not an illness or a disease. Nor were they a lump or a case. They were not even patients. They were frightened, sick people who had come to us seeking solutions to their problems. Our primary responsibility was to listen, understand, and make them feel at ease. He was totally involved with them and their problems, and he expected us to do the same. His Aussie accent was terribly confusing as he pronounced A as I. When he told us to wait in I-ward, we waited for him in I-ward while he looked for us in A-ward. When he discharged a patient, he told him, *You can go home today.* The patient was aghast, having heard, *You can go home to die!*

I remember accompanying him to visit patients in their homes to see how they fared after being discharged. Completely at home, the Australian surgeon would sit cross-legged in their thatched mud-floor houses and share their meal. He always took one of us with him, and we learnt more from those visits than we ever did in a classroom. Dr Garlick had a training board with hooks and sutures that we practised on. We fumbled with granny knots that would not hold even as he taught us surgical knots that we practised for hours until we could do them in our sleep. To teach us the art of scrubbing meticulously before surgery, he would smear car grease all the way up to our elbows and make us scrub until we were squeaky clean. He was never impatient, and it seemed as if our surgical training was the only thing on his mind. He encouraged us to conduct examinations and procedures on each other, stopping short only at the pelvic and rectal examinations. Dr Garlick was an unforgettable teacher who taught by example.

Dr D Paranjothy's clinics

Dr Paranjothy introduced us to obstetrics and gynaecology. I do not know if I can describe her 3-D personality in words. A diminutive lady, whose white doctor's coat dwarfed her, walking down the corridors of the hospital with purpose in every step was only the tip of the iceberg. Dr Paranjothy was omnipresent. You looked up, and she was there, completely and totally committed to her patients and students. I doubt if she ever went home.

Every woman who crossed the half-swing door into the Gynae OPD left only after a pelvic examination, even if she had come in with a headache. That was one of Dr Paranjothy's many rules. *They will complain about a headache or something totally unrelated because they are shy. You have to get past that*, she would say. In her book, every patient in her reproductive years was pregnant unless proven otherwise, and every pregnancy was an ectopic, a pregnancy outside the uterus, unless proven otherwise.

One day, a young woman came in with a chronic vaginal infection that was refractory to treatment. It was draining her, and she had gone from pillar to post seeking a cure. Dr Paranjothy examined her, prescribed some vaginal pessaries, and told us to explain the insertion of the pessary to the patient as she moved on to examine the patient in the next cubicle. Vaginal pessaries were fairly new, and women in rural India were definitely not a tactile species in the 1960s. Most of them were absolutely clueless about their anatomy. I drew a diagram that looked like a game of knots and crosses in the margin of the chart, and I showed her precisely where she had to insert it. *Insert it into this one*, I said, pointing with my pencil, *Not the other one,* I said, repeatedly circling the correct aperture.

The patient hid her face behind her sari and giggled. Seeing that I was getting nowhere with my class on female anatomy, someone else took over and explained the basics to the patient again, even as the patient continued to giggle. Finally, one of the girls had a brilliant idea. *Maybe we could teach her to insert it like a tampon,* she said. Turning to the patient, she said, *Wash your hand with soap and water. Put your left foot on a stool. Pick up the pessary with the thumb and index finger of your right hand, and insert it in here,* she said, pointing to my diagram of knots and crosses. The patient nodded as if she had finally understood where to insert it.

We thought that we had seen the last of her when she picked up her prescription and left. Just as we were leaving for lunch, the patient appeared at the door and stood there with her arms akimbo. There were a zillion people around us as she looked over everyone's heads straight at Dr Paranjothy. Waving the packet of pessaries in the air, she asked, *Ye Ma, oru kaal nakali mela thooki vechi sapidava? Madam, should I put one foot on the stool and swallow it?* So much for my stick diagram of knots and crosses!

Dr Paranjothy would be called for consultations by other specialities. Most male doctors had a morbid fear of anything OG-logical in nature, and they would swiftly send off for a Gynaec consult claiming that the female pelvis and the organs of reproduction in lady-land were a mystery to man and beast. One day, I accompanied her when she was called to examine a young woman who had been admitted to the neurology ward with a right-sided hemiplegia. The patient and her family had been to several hospitals and had used up most of their resources. CMC Vellore was their last hope. The patient's chart said that the twenty-four-year-old had a living child, aged three.

There were no other details except that she had undergone a D&C for an incomplete abortion four months ago.

Dr Paranjothy was a completely different personality when she was with her patients. Her rare smiles were reserved only for patients whom she examined with an air of experience and confidence, a combination that patients found instantly comforting. Reassured, the patient filled in the history, helping Dr Paranjothy join the dots. When asked, the patient recounted that she had passed grape-like tissue during her second pregnancy, a pathognomonic sign of a molar pregnancy. She was taken to a local hospital for a D&C and later discharged with vitamins, words of wisdom about family planning, and no date for a follow-up. She developed weakness of the muscles on her right side two months later. With her meticulous history taking, Dr Paranjothy diagnosed a molar pregnancy, which had led to a choriocarcinoma that was caused by malignant changes in the cells that form the placenta. In this case it had metastasised to the brain and resulted in hemiplegia – paralysis of her right upper and lower limbs. In minutes she had the diagnosis at the bedside, without any expensive imaging, scan, or MRI. *The patient will always lead you to a diagnosis if you listen,* she said, turning to me. *Eyes and ears first, everything else afterwards.*

The labour room posting

As final year students, we were required to submit a record of twenty normal deliveries that we had conducted on our own, before our final exam. Posted to the labour room in batches of four in what was considered a punishment posting, we were held as hostages in the attic above the labour room. We had to be there all the time, and there was no question of leaving until we had seen the mothers-to-be through all three stages of labour, replete with contraceptive advice or intervention. This was completely non-negotiable in Dr Paranjothy's book. The attic above the labour room was a dreary room with a single window on one wall and a stuffy bathroom in a corner. The four beds in the centre of the room covered with grey-hospital-sheets-that-once-were-white were kept deliberately uncomfortable so that no medical student born of flesh and blood could sleep through a summons from the labour room.

We were expected to go to sleep with our saris perfectly pinned and pleated on our person to save time. Our white coat, slippers, and stethoscopes were placed strategically at the foot end of the bed, close enough to be grabbed en route to the labour room. No one cared if you had not brushed your teeth or powdered your nose, but all hell would break loose if your nails were long and lacquered or if your hair was not knotted, tied up, and out of harm's way. A bell connected us to the labour room downstairs. When it rang, we would tumble down in various stages of disarray to receive the patient, with or without the nurses, in the labour room. Only when we started interacting with the nurses did we begin to appreciate the pivotal role they play in patient care. Why they spend more time caring for the patients than doctors ever did!

Many of the patients, young and frightened, admitted for their first delivery as unbooked cases, had never visited a hospital before and they found hospitalisation intimidating. The women preferred a lady doctor to attend to them when they went into labour, so the boys in our batch had an easy run. They were molly-coddled by the lady professors and got away scot-free because the faculty actually believed that none of the boys would ever stray into lady-land to specialise in anything remotely OG-logical. The nurses would prep the cases for the boys, and hand them over on a platter with the promise to help if they needed anything. This usually meant that the nurses did everything for the boys, and the boys did practically nothing, much to our combined chagrin.

The girls, on the other hand, had to receive the patients the moment they entered the labour room, prep them, shave them, give them a high, hot enema, and hold their hand as they waddled to and from the bathroom to empty their bladder.

Since no one expected the boys to do Ob/Gyn anyway, Dr Paranjothy felt they did not need to waste their time. They could go and read in the library or go and stuff their faces in the canteen, which is what they did. In the 1960s, everyone presumed that every female medical student had only one career option: to end up as an obstetrician/gynaecologist.

This preposterous gender slant was perpetuated not because the girls were not smart enough to pursue other branches of medicine, but because women of that era would never part their legs to be examined by a male doctor. They would rather die in childbirth and take their unborn children with them than be examined by a strange man. The boys in our class who were posted to the labour room would waltz in and out sniggering, and it took every ounce of our good upbringing not to punch their noses. This meant that the girls were trained extremely well, and as predicted, none of our class boys specialised in lady-land.

The dreaded VF

Dr Paranjothy had several rules in the labour room that had to be followed to a tee. *When the patient goes into labour, students,* she would say, *make sure she is well hydrated. See that she empties her bowels and bladder at regular intervals.* This was easier said than done. When a patient is in labour, and her uterine contractions have blocked out all reason, the last thing she wants to hear is anyone else's advice about her bodily functions, especially when none of us, as medical students, barely out of our teens, could speak with authority on the subject. *As if they know*, they would scoff.

The birth canal, the bladder, and the rectum are in close proximity to one another. The bladder is aligned in front of the birth canal. The descending head of the baby could press against the bladder and cause retention of urine. As labour progressed, the patient would find it difficult to void. If this goes on for a long time, the prolonged pressure of the baby's head on the mother's bladder can cause the tissue between the mother's bladder and vagina to necrotise and slough, creating a fistula, an unnatural passage between the bladder and the vagina, the dreaded vesicovaginal fistula (VVF). Normally, urine produced continuously in the kidney flows to the bladder to be stored before voiding. With a defect in the bladder, the urine cannot be stored, causing a continuous dribble of urine from the bladder to the vagina and down a woman's inner legs for the rest of her life, sentencing her to life as a social outcast with no love life to write home about. VVFs do not heal spontaneously. They require complicated surgical repair, sometimes in expensive stages, often out of reach of women in rural areas. These are precisely the women who are prone to developing VVFs because they are often unbooked cases with all the complications of obstructed labour, seeking late help.

When she was in the labour room, Dr Paranjothy made sure that all the patients voided spontaneously. Catheterisation carried the risk of infection and was done only when there was no other option. *Students, go and open the tap in the bathroom,* she would say, *Make sure it's half-open. The sound of dripping water will encourage the patient to pass. You'll see.* She would be right, of course. The patient would eventually pass urine. The only problem was that the rest of the bladders in the labour room would also come under the influence of the dripping tap. We would run upstairs cross-legged to the attic, as fast as we could with our bladders reaching our clavicles.

As medical students in the early 1960s, we saw many VVFs that could be sniffed a mile away. As PGs in the late 1970s, we did not. Fortunately, with increasing awareness, better antenatal care, and good obstetric practices reaching the rural population, VVFs are now seen only occasionally, if at all.

Sister Victor and the miracle of birth

Learning about the anatomy and physiology of the *Passage and the Passenger* between the covers of a book or in a classroom was absolutely fine. Watching it in high definition as a 3-D film in real life, accompanied by adrenaline-driven audio-visuals, was entirely another thing. I remember the first delivery I witnessed. I was assisting Sister Victor, the senior sister in charge of the labour room, the mother figure we gravitated to when we were in trouble. She was highly experienced and so very senior that I think she may even have been present when I was born in CMC, twenty years before my posting as a medical student to the Attic.

My first patient was a young girl, Latha, who was around my age. This was her first pregnancy, and her husband, who had another wife and a family of grown-up children, was fifteen years older than her. He was in the corridor outside the labour room, waiting to hear the cry of their firstborn. The corridor was not a waiting room, and there were no seats for the patient's relatives. This did not stop them from standing or sitting outside, huddled in groups until they were sent packing by the hospital security, only to return later when the coast was clear. Communication between the patient and her relatives waiting anxiously in the corridor happened only through a ventilator positioned above the patient's bed. Sometimes the pregnant patient would climb up on the railing of her bed to get close to the ventilator when a fall would have been disastrous. Latha, who blamed her husband for her present predicament, was in no mood to risk her life climbing up to whisper sweet nothings through the ventilator.

I helped the nurse prep Latha, and I stayed with her as she progressed in labour, plying her with fluids to keep her well hydrated. She was not interested in eating or drinking anything. All she wanted to do was go to the toilet. She refused to use the bedpan we offered and would insist on dragging herself to the toilets at the end of the corridor, stopping to watch the action in each cubicle, with eyes as big as saucers. She was not bothered that the green hospital gown she wore was open at the back with half-done ties, revealing her gluteal cleft. At the zenith of her contractions, modesty was the last thing on her mind.

We had been talking, and I knew that she was frightened. When she was ready to deliver and bear down, Sister Victor was called. She seemed to have everything under control when she started explaining the miracle of birth to me. A lovely person with a matronly figure, Sister Victor was perched precariously on a rotating steel stool at the foot end of the cold, steel labour room cot. Latha was in the lithotomy position, ready for the birth of her baby, with her legs up in the air, pulled apart, and strapped into stirrups. A million trainee nurses were holding her down and encouraging her to push. *Push, push, Mukku-ma, Mukku-ma, Mukku*, they bellowed.

Unfrazzled, Sister Victor continued to explain the miracle of birth to me as I stood riveted, a few steps behind her. Periodically, she would lift the green sheets that covered Latha's nether regions and peer in. I could not concentrate on anything she was saying from her rotating stool as I was too distracted by everything happening around me. Suddenly, there was a *swoooooosh* sound, and there was water all over the floor as Latha's membranes ruptured and the amniotic fluid gushed out.

The ward aides, standing close, swooped down and mopped the floor in turns. All I heard was the terrified screams and grunts that were coming from Latha's head end. I felt so sorry for her. I could feel this huge lump growing in my throat. I felt her pain, and I felt as if every scream from her was coming from me even though my mouth appeared closed. Suddenly, I saw a tuft of curly black hair appear, and I saw Sister Victor reach for a pair of sterile scissors, poised to do an episiotomy on Latha, an incision that would help her deliver the head of her baby. That was the final straw. I heard Sister Victor's voice from a distance, *Susie, are you watching?*

There was no answer from Susie.

Susie had fled. Susie had run out of the labour room.

Taught by example

We were blessed to have professors and teachers who taught by example. On meagre salaries they never complained about, they walked through the wards dressed in simple white cottons and open sandals. The ladies were impeccably dressed in starched cotton saris that they wore pinned and pleated, often through hot and humid days. The senior professors and heads of departments considered teaching undergraduate medical students their primary duty. If there were interesting cases in the ward, they would call out to any of us students in sight and show us the cases, taking impromptu clinics for us. The more we hung around the wards, the more we saw and the more we learnt. Most of what we learnt did not come from our prescribed textbooks; it came from the patients we saw in clinics. Most of the common diseases we met during our clinical years had a face, a name, an anecdote, and a memory of a committed teacher who taught us by example.

Edgar Dale said, *We remember ten per cent of what we read, twenty per cent of what we hear, thirty per cent of what we see, fifty per cent of what we see and hear, seventy per cent of what we discuss with others, eighty per cent of what we personally experience, and ninety per cent of what we teach others.*

Infectious diseases posting, Madras

We attended clinics at the Infectious Diseases Hospital in Tondiarpet, in Madras, to see cases on grand rounds. The entire trip was an eye-opener for us as we had never seen a government-run hospital before. We were astounded by the footfall in the hospital. Sick patients milled around doctors and nurses in dusty rooms and corridors with hardly any privacy. The queues at the pharmacy were serpentine, and the admissions in the wards spilt onto mats on the floor, replete with IV infusions on flow. We saw more cases of cholera and typhoid in a few hours at the Infectious Diseases Hospital than we had seen in all our clinical years at CMC. The numbers were mind-boggling. We even saw a case of smallpox, the first and last case we would ever see. A disfigured young woman covered in cruel, infectious scabs lay huddled on the cold floor of the hospital veranda, a visual I see with enormous clarity so many years later.

Viva in Madras

We took our written exams in Vellore and travelled to Madras for our practical exams and viva, to be held in one of the government colleges, usually Madras Medical College or

Stanley Medical College. Our papers were sent to the examiners who were posted at various colleges to evaluate us. Our passing depended on us independently clearing the written exam, the practical test, and the viva. We were allowed to camp in one of the hostels for the days that we had our viva. I remember sleeping on the table tennis table in the games room of one of the hostels. In unfamiliar surroundings and at a distinct disadvantage, we wandered around bewildered and lost.

The students from the local colleges knew all the specimens that had been picked for the exams. Hearing their discussions, our morale would plummet further. On D-Day, we would muster all the courage and confidence that we did not have to go in and answer the viva to the best of our ability, describing what we saw, as it was, nothing more and nothing less. This was precisely what was expected of us as undergraduates, though we did not know it then, as we stood out like sore thumbs in our starched, pleated cotton saris and worried expressions.

On my way to Madras for my final year practical exams, I met Titu Thomas, one of our seniors, a registrar in medicine. He showed me a case of hydro pneumothorax, when air and fluid enter the pleural space. We had only read about it; I had never seen a case before. He went over the history and findings with me while I examined the patient. When I reported to Madras for my medicine clinical exam, I was astounded when my long case turned out to be hydro pneumothorax, almost as if the patient had travelled on the bus with me. Only the face of the patient was different. I could hear Titu's voice going over all the findings, including the succussion splash, and my heart sang. If Titu had not shown me the case, I would have missed all the findings and flunked my finals. There are no accidents in life, and this is just one of the many occasions in my life that reaffirmed my faith that no matter what lay ahead, the

Almighty went before me, and He never left my side.

Internship
Before we knew it, we had passed our final year exams and become interns. Responsibility was a fourteen-letter word in a twenty-four-hour day for an intern at the bottom of the pile.

We had to clerk cases, send investigations, collect results, prepare discharge summaries, and be in five different places all at once. Duty nights were a sleepless blur. Meals were a *rush 'n' gobble affair,* and *leave* a dirty five-letter word allowed only in case of death or disaster. At the end of twelve months, we could have survived anything anywhere.

Medicine
I did my medicine internship with Dr TS Koshy, easily one of the kindest professors on the faculty. Gentle and soft-spoken, with a shy smile on his face, Dr TSK was a man of few words. On rounds, his kind eyes and shy smile seemed to soothe anxious patients when they were frightened and confused.

It was a pleasure to go on rounds with him. He never lost his cool, never threw tantrums, and never got angry with us though he could get a point across effectively and sweetly when he had to with a smile. He never needed to yell or discipline us to get the best out of us. And his patients loved him!

Surgery
My surgical posting was in surgery unit two with Dr Fenn, who had an impressive list of rich and famous celebrities that he operated upon. Some were glamorous stars from the film world, some were fiery personalities from the political world, and some were giants from the sporting world. No two grand rounds were ever the same, nor were any two days in the theatre.

We learnt to expect the unexpected when Dr Fenn, *Chief* as he was affectionately called, was around.

One day I was sitting on the floor in the operation theatre writing up a discharge summary when I heard his baritone rising in crescendo. I thought Dr Fenn was singing in the theatre. He was not singing. He was having an epiphany moment with a scrub nurse who had just handed him the wrong instrument for the third time. A second later, the scalpel flew across the sanitised floor as it left Dr Fenn's clenched fist, sending us running for cover.

Ob/Gyn

I did my Ob/Gyn posting with Dr Prabhavathy Kunders, a HOD with legendary surgical skills. Like Dr Paranjothy, she too was extremely lenient with the boys in our batch but extremely tough with the girls, which annoyed us intensely. As Dr Kunders' unit had all the *Who's Who* of society, we were lucky if we got to shine the light for her during an episiotomy. If the light we held trailed out of her operating zone, she would look up and ask us whether we thought she was doing neurosurgery in the labour room! Once, she agreed to an expat husband's unusual request to be present at his wife's delivery. In the 1960s and 1970s most husbands never entered the labour room. Dr Kunders was aghast when the husband arrived with his high-tech camera and a blinding spotlight to record the event for posterity. Unselfconscious, and completely in sync with nature, he kept encouraging his wife to relax *to the maximum* in his best French accent. An acutely embarrassed and uncomfortable Dr Kunders was extremely relieved when she was saved by the bell and called away to an emergency, leaving her assistants to conduct the grand finale. When the nurses expressed the excess milk from the patient to prevent engorgement of the breast, the husband collected it religiously without fail. All this *doing what comes naturally* was too much for the ward's young nurses and junior doctors who collapsed in piles of giggles in the corridor.

Community medicine

I did a twelve-week rural posting at the CSI hospital in Nagari. When the CMC van dropped me off at the hospital, I was taken to meet Dr Beard, the expat medical superintendent, a missionary from England. Everyone in Nagari called her *Beard Amma*, which translated meant *the bearded mother*. She was, in actual fact, the complete opposite of this incongruous nickname. Slim and tall, Dr Beard was a beautiful woman without a hint of fuzz on her face. She looked like an angel with her peaches and cream complexion untouched by the harsh Indian sun. She covered distances with a few light steps that I found hard to match as I ran alongside her to the theatre for a Caesarean section.

After scrubbing, I went in to find her standing on the left of the patient. I was a bit confused as the surgeon usually stands on the right side. Thinking that we were both going to assist some other doctor, I went and stood beside her on the left side. She waved me round to the right side and said, *Start*, as she handed me the scalpel. *Me?* I squeaked incredulously. In my surgery and ob/gyn postings at CMC, I was delirious if I got to hold a retractor for an operation. I could not believe that she was expecting me to lay the incision. I was so happy I thought I would burst.

The Nagari experience was simply outstanding as we did everything hands-on. BDR Paul, a senior alumnus, loved and respected by the whole village, was doing his mission bond at Nagari. He and Dr Beard let us handle difficult cases while staying within calling distance. Our learning graph soared with confidence, and gratitude, with every day we spent at Nagari.

The cases were intriguing and unpredictable, each one more exciting than the last. Sometimes it was a woman exhausted after a prolonged labour. Sometimes it was a septic abortion - the handiwork of an untrained local midwife who tried to terminate an unwanted pregnancy under unsterile conditions, resulting in heinous complications. Curious objects, blunt and sharp, lay waiting to be recovered from the patient's anatomy. These instruments, abandoned in lady-land, were objects that were inserted to start or complete an abortion.

Sometimes the bullock cart trundled in babies with dehydration or seizures. There were snake and scorpion bites galore in a countryside where people walked barefoot and shared the environment with flora and fauna. Sometimes it was an elderly citizen with pneumonia, a broken bone after a fall, or a nasty road transport accident. I remember a drunken driver, too inebriated to make sense, who kept looking at the lifeless man lying still on the next bed, totally confused that there was only one corpse lying next to him. He kept urging us to go back and find the other two that he was sure he had mowed down.

I was truly sorry to leave Nagari at the end of three months. Later, when I worked in isolation in Nepal and Bhutan, my early days at Nagari with Dr Beard helped me surge forward in confidence as I faced the quagmires that baffled me.

Is there a doctor on the train?

My hands-on training in Nagari came in useful on one of my trips on the Southern Railway. I was going to Kerala with my Mum's youngest sister, my Aunt *Ponnocho,* who was visiting from Singapore on a short holiday. We were in the second-class AC compartment and had just settled down in our berths when the ticket collector came through asking if there was a doctor on board.

I did not have to answer. My aunt, bursting with pride, piped up. *Yes yes. My niece is a doctor. She has just passed her MBBS. My niece, this one... this one... She is a doctor,* she said, pushing a reluctant me forward.

The ticket collector looked me up and down as I sat there in a skirt, a blouse, slippers, and two pigtails. I do not think he was very impressed. His look implied, *Has she really finished college?* However, since he was desperate, he had no choice but to settle for what he got. *There is a lady in labour in the ladies' compartment,* he said. *Jolarpet is another hour away, and I don't think she will last till the train reaches the station. Do you think you can help?* Before I could open my mouth, my aunt piped up again. *Of course she can, lah. She has conducted so many deliveries*, she said with a flamboyant sweep of her hand. Swelling with pride, she pushed me off the berth and sent me with the ticket collector.

When I got to the ladies compartment, a green cotton sari had been pulled across the section as a makeshift screen. Lifting the sari, I went in. Lying on the left lower berth with her legs towards the closed window was a middle-aged lady clearly in established labour. I had no antiseptic to wash or scrub with. What I did have was an unopened bottle of my favourite perfume, *Charlie*, in my handbag, which my aunt had just brought me from Singapore. No gloves. No drapes. No stirrups. No time to think. Dousing myself with *Charlie*, my training kicked in. Wasting no time, I supported the patient's multiparous, lax and much-stretched perineum as she bore down and delivered a beautiful baby girl who gulped for air and cried at birth with a perfect Apgar score. Everyone in the compartment cheered when they heard the baby cry. A quick check confirmed that there was no tear and that the mother's perineum was intact. Meanwhile, the women in the compartment who were older than me and definitely more experienced in matters of the world were tripping over themselves, trying to be helpful. They offered me all sorts of objects, sharp and blunt, to cut the cord once the baby was delivered. Pretending to be selectively deaf, I held on without turning around. I was not going to cut the cord in a crowded, obviously unsterile, ladies compartment on a moving Southern Railway train. *No way! Especially when Jolarpet was just down the track.* I waited until the cord stopped pulsating and delivered the placenta while it was still attached to the bawling infant by an intact, uncut cord. *No cut, no sepsis, no tetanus*, I thought to myself.

The co-passengers in the compartment that had doubled up spontaneously as a labour room were unbelievably generous. Seeing the woman cold and drenched in amniotic fluid and blood, they opened up their bags and offered her clean clothes to change into in a touching gesture. Jolarpet station had been alerted, and paramedics were waiting in attendance as the train drew up onto the platform. The mother, the neonate with the intact cord and placenta were transferred to a Southern Railway stretcher and taken off the train. As she was lowered onto the stretcher, the mother reached out, held my hand, and thanked me. *I am going to name her after you*, she said with a wan smile. I felt really good. Being a doctor was all right, I thought to myself as Mrs Holloway and the white coat flashed in my brain!

When we reached Thiruvalla, my aunt rang my Mum and told her that I had delivered a baby on a moving train. My Mum did some sympathetic swelling in Singapore and told my aunt to buy me anything I wanted when we went shopping!

Graduation day

Soon it was graduation day. *Would a cap, a gown, and a piece of paper reflect even a fraction of the transformation we had undergone in the six years we had spent at CMC?* we wondered. We were not the gawky teenagers who had been dropped off in the sunken garden of the college in front of the chapel. Our lives had changed indefinably as we morphed into the seniors we had admired as freshers. We had filled up and filled out as we matured in ways seen and unseen. We had been pruned and polished as we met birth, death, and disease in the corridors of life. We had rubbed shoulders with patients from all walks of life - the good, the bad, the ugly, the rich, the poor, the haves, and the have-nots.

We had seen families pawn all that they had to bring one member of the family for treatment We had seen the same families take their dead home covered in a white sheet when the treatment had been too little, too late, failed or when death was inevitable. When hope changed to despair, unsurmountable financial debt, and ruination. We had seen abortions and infertility cases in adjacent cubicles in the same OPD. Wanted babies and unwanted babies had arrived simultaneously, ignoring pomp and circumstance. We had learnt to be players in a team and follow orders as internes at the bottom of the pile.

Life was definitely not black and white. Sometimes it was not even grey. We were poised to take on the world, though a tad apprehensive. Our names had acquired extra letters, two in front and four at the end. We were doctors and carried the weight of expectation on our shoulders and the cold realisation of a frail humanity in our hearts and soul.

The CMC graduation ceremony is unforgettable.

Lined up in ascending order of height, the final year boys in college blazers and the final year girls in white saris proudly carry a spectacular jasmine chain several metres long on their shoulders as a guard of honour for the graduates and the faculty in their regalia to walk through. *The Graduation Chimes*, a majestic mix of Western classical music strung together aesthetically, is timed and tuned to a tee to match the measured steps the guard of honour takes from the verdant grounds to the dais of the Scudder Auditorium. The Graduation Chimes introduced by Dr P Zac start with the *Trumpet Voluntary* and end with the *Triumphal March* of the grand opera *Aida* by Verdi. An emotional Pavlovian experience, it is conditioned to evoke nostalgic goosebumps and a wondrous reminder of the most important walk in a young medical graduate's life.

Robed and capped in our new clothes, we walked down the jasmine chain of honour. Goosebumps came and goosebumps went with every step of the Graduation Chimes as we were ushered to our seats in the front rows of the auditorium. Decades later, even as I write this, I can feel the goosebumps as I recall the awe I felt in October 1970 at my graduation ceremony in the Scudder Auditorium in CMC Vellore. Only when the faculty is seated on the dais does the Graduation Chimes stop. A few minutes later, the piano plays the first few bars of the college song, and the auditorium rustles as everyone stands to sing the college song *Girded Round By the Strong Ageless Mountains*, with a lump in their throats.

When our names were called out, we walked up to the dais to receive our diploma. Our hearts pounded as blood rushed to parts of our bodies we did not even know we had. Nothing this grand or important had ever happened to us in our whole lives. We stood up as a batch and took the Hippocratic Oath in collective reverence, in the hushed auditorium as a rite of passage to go out into the world and practise medicine. I wonder if we understood the enormity of all that we had solemnly promised to follow. Did we have any idea of what lay ahead for us?

The alumni

At the end of our internship, we became alumni, old students of the Christian Medical College Vellore. *Old* being the operative word as the years rolled by. CMC alumni are never referred to as ex-students. This would suggest a relationship in the past tense, when we left college. Ours never did. In addition to our medical degrees, we were given alumni friendships to treasure. When the alumni grew into a prolific gene pool and threatened to disintegrate into a disorderly database, burying nuggets of pride and valuable information, Dr P Zac dared to dream of an alumni directory. Assisted by Dr Molly Bhanu and Dr Grace Chandi, he meticulously traced the alumni across the globe, collated their contact information, professional milestones, awards, accolades, and the names of their current spouse and progeny.

Once completed, the directory even had the names of the alumni in heaven! It took Dr P Zac and his team twenty tedious years to publish the first silver-and-blue alumni directory, which now serves as a travel advisory, a global *Airbnb*, and a compass to reunite lost friends and rekindle memories of a time when life was simple, friendships were easy, and one walked on water for the other. An invaluable diplomatic portal, its sensitive marital data is current enough to prevent people from inadvertently dropping the names of old flames at reunions, saving discomfiture all around. Not everyone married their college crushes.

Alumni reunions

Every year, over the second weekend in August, the college hosts a reunion when alumni from all over the world meet in

Vellore. Alumni from batches five years apart, e.g. fifty, fifty-five, sixty, and so on, are invited as chief guests.

The reunion starts on a Friday in the Norman Auditorium at the hospital, when distinguished alumni address the student body in an interactive meeting, to inspire the current medical students. The speakers range from distinguished heads of premier institutes in India or overseas in smart suits and gleaming shoes, to alumni in open sandals working resolutely in resource-poor areas, often as the only healthcare givers for miles around. These contrasts may appear to be sharp to the untrained eye, but they are really two sides of the same coin, each bringing their own brand of courage, charisma, and dignity to the dais.

Dr Ida Scudder's dream was to train competent, committed doctors for the villages in all the remote parts of India where healthcare had not made tracks. Young medical students at the crossroads of their lives who are debating career options got a chance to listen to someone who had once sat on the same benches with the same aspirations and dreams—an erstwhile medical student who was now out in the world doing a hands-on job and enjoying it either in a milieu of plenty or paucity.

Vespers in the chapel is a moving mix of alumni, both young and old, renewing tradition. Fresh graduates are welcomed by senior alumni and given unlit candles that super seniors light for them, a symbolic rite of passage. A senior alumnus from one of the special batches, someone who had once sat in the chapel as a fresh graduate years ago, delivers the sermon.

The highlight of the evening is the poignant roll call of the names of the alumni who died in that particular year. As the names are called, a friend or classmate walks up to the altar, bathed in the soft dim light of the chapel, to light a candle in loving remembrance of the deceased alumnus. Memories come tumbling down. Eyes are moist. A smile escapes when a prank or escapade is remembered. The world may forget you, but CMC never forgets her alumni. The service closes with the sevenfold amen that Dr Bob Carman and Dr Poonnoose Mathew taught the choir to sing *acapella*, and the alumni leave charged to face the challenges ahead.

Saturday dinner with the familiar Biryani at the Scudder Auditorium is followed by an evening of entertainment, mainly a mix of silly fun and serious talent ending with a Sri Lankan Baila, with everyone dancing in the foyer to mark the end of another annual alumni weekend.

With back-to-back formal programmes and informal catching-up sessions, the emotional weekend chalks up sleepless nights. Every aged and creaky joint is ready to go home by Sunday when the tender farewells start. Alumni friendships are a legacy. Vintage grey hair, a pound, a fold or two, a wrinkle here or there, only adds to the highs of happy reunions. Apparently normal sane adults can be reduced to screeching adolescents with astonishing ease. Incredulous kids are left speechless and apologising amongst themselves for their parents aberrant and juvenile behaviour.

These friendships can be picked up anytime, anywhere from where they are left off. The unique and legendary bond shared by the CMC alumni is a legacy, a blessing in ways more than one. When the *do-you-remember-whens* take over, the *in-between-years* do not matter or count. CMC alumni include state-of-the-art researchers to doctors without borders to dedicated clinicians working tirelessly with bare essentials in resource-poor settings. Sometimes this can create invisible trammels when batchmates meet many years later away from the wooden benches they sat on side by side in college until the memories of their college days takeover to cut through snob and snobbery. CMC takes pride in all its alumni, no matter where they work, how much they earn or how much they are worth. It is the spirit of CMC, reflected in the alumnus, that counts wherever he or she is called to work.

Postgraduate studies

I returned to academia to complete my postgraduate studies in two completely unrelated fields in two different continents, two kids and ten years apart. After our posting in Bhutan, Sam and I went to the UK for our postgraduate studies, leaving our kids, Rekha and Anish, with my parents in Madras. The plan was that once we had settled into our jobs, we would take the children. Unfortunately, this did not happen.

A couple of months after we went to the UK, while I was preparing for part one of the membership exam to the Royal College of Obstetricians & Gynaecologists (MRCOG), my Dad suffered two consecutive heart attacks in Madras, leaving my Mum in her seventies struggling to cope on her own. I returned to India for my PG studies in Vellore to be near them and visit them on weekends, leaving Sam to fend for himself in England with a copy of a Tarla Dalal cookbook. For two years, we could not get the equation right, and the four of us, Sam, Rekha, Anish, and I, were in three different cities.

DGO

The Diploma in Gynaecology and Obstetrics (DGO) was a two-year programme at CMC. Dr SX Charles, the HOD of the OG department, was one of the earliest male gynaecologists in CMC to foray into a completely female-dominated speciality. He motivated all of us, and me in particular, to pass our exams in the first attempt. Dr Prabha Jairaj and Dr Bala trained us in the labour room, outpatient clinics, and in the operation theatre, to stay focused even as we juggled sanity and skill.

When I came back to CMC to do my DGO, Joyce Ponnaiya, Gracy Thomas, and Vanaja Verghese were doing their postgraduate studies. Gracy and Vanaja were my seniors from college. Joyce was my classmate. I would never have survived my DGO were it not for the three of them and others like Lakshmi Seshadri, a young bride from Coimbatore; Padmini Jasper; and many others who were doing their PG at the same time. Together we formed a protective band of friends to survive. We all had only one agenda, to finish the course as soon as possible and go home to our families. Nothing else mattered. Ob/Gyn was a hands-on, adrenaline-driven speciality, where we learned as we worked. The harder we worked, the more we learned. On reflection, after those two years of rigorous training, we were tough and resilient enough to survive anything, anywhere.

Our only recreation was the movies in town. Leaving behind the day with its ups and downs, the PGs who were free, would pile into open-top cycle rickshaws and ride to the cinema theatres in town. We never missed a single movie that came to town. It did not matter if the movie was a hit or a flop or if it was in English, a regional language or vernacular. Somebody in the group would translate, and sometimes the running commentary would end up being more hilarious than the movie itself. Sometimes we fell asleep, exhausted and lulled to sleep by the cool air conditioning and the darkened theatre, needing to be nudged awake when the movie ended. Movies gave us a chance to forget the day's woes for a few hours in the comfort of the air conditioning.

Rat... rat... rat

On one occasion, there was a group of roadside Romeos sitting behind our row of seats. As the projector whirred on, it became increasingly evident that they were more interested in the women in front of them than they were in the movie. They kept passing lewd comments and smacking their lips. Some leaned forward, breathing lecherously down our necks, bent on being obnoxious. One of them, an uncouth youth who was more adventurous than the others, slid his sweaty paw between the seats and pinched one of our seniors right on her exposed midriff between her sari and blouse. The poor unsuspecting guy had no clue that you never mess with the likes of this particular senior, who shall remain nameless, unless you were prepared for *Rani of Jhansi* to rise from the ashes. She was as spunky as she was beautiful, with a spirit to match her curvy silhouette. Absolutely fearless, she stood up, whipped around with her slipper in hand, and whacked him straight across his surprised face. *How dare you!* she hissed as she flayed him with stinging slaps. *Take that... And that.*

The youth was stunned and mortified. This was a response he had never ever encountered before. Beads of sweat gleamed on his crumpled face as the projector light shone into the darkened theatre hall. He was used to eve-teasing timid girls who either suffered it all in silence or moved to another part of the theatre, but none of them had ever spun around to attack him. He was caught completely off guard, and his jaw dropped in shock and horror. Mortified, and in an attempt to regain his dignity and composure, he squeaked, *It's a rat. It's a rat. A rat must have bitten you... rat... rat.* He bent down, pretending to look for the elusive rat. This only incensed the lady further, who whacked him some more as she yelled, *Rat? Did you say rat? You are the rat! Nee thaan Da perichali! You're the big, Fat bandicoot!*

The back row emptied in a matter of minutes while the rest of us cheered. I suspect it was many moons before they annoyed anybody again.

The tragedies

The cases that came to the casualty after mismanaged manipulations outside were horrendous. The objects used by quacks to induce septic abortions in the early 1970s could be anything from a knitting needle to a wood apple, each object more bizarre than the next. It was inconceivable for an unwed mother to raise a child with dignity in the early 1970s. Contraceptives were not available as over-the-counter prescriptions, and sex education was a dirty word people never used in public, least of all in schools or colleges. The gynae OPD in CMC would occasionally throw up the *odd* abdominal tumour with a viable heartbeat, an unwanted pregnancy.

One particular girl I will never forget was Usha, a beautiful sixteen-year-old with a charming smile, long black hair, and mischief dancing in her eyes, a mere child in so many ways. She studied in a convent and had never left home. No sleepovers. No excursions. No contact with the opposite sex or so the parents thought.

What she did have, however, was her father's cousin, who had come to Vellore in search of a job. One thing led to another, and she became prey to his advances as they started meeting surreptitiously whenever her parents stepped out for the odd chore. Clueless about contraception, she soon became pregnant. When she missed a couple of periods, the boy panicked and returned to his village.

Alone and frightened, she watched as her belly grew imperceptibly. One morning, when she started having abdominal cramps, her mother brought her to the clinic. What they described as a stomach ache was confirmed as a twenty-four-week pregnancy. Paralysed with fear, the mother begged for an abortion. She said that they could not bring an illegitimate child into their world. Her father would beat Usha to a pulp and then kill her. Unfortunately, a mid-trimester termination would have been dangerous. We advised her to go and talk to her father. Usha and her mother left the clinic, and an uneasy calm settled among us. None of us looked at each other or talked about it after they left. We just felt uncomfortable. Perhaps we knew what would happen.

Three days later, I got a bleep from casualty. When I parted the green curtain that separated the cubicles, I saw Usha lying limp and pale on the bed while her mother wept inconsolably into a towel. Usha had been brought in minutes earlier in a moribund state. They had started a drip and sent off her investigations with a request for a pint of blood. She was lying in a pool of blood, and the pair of broken bloodstained knitting needles and the bloodstained glove that lay between her legs spoke volumes. Slowly, we got the history from the mother.

They never told the father. They found a quack on the other side of town working out of a back room in her home. The quack introduced her well-travelled knitting needles into Usha's vagina with her legs pulled wide apart with no anaesthesia. The rest was history. When Usha started bleeding profusely, and as her screams became fainter and fainter, the quack and her bouncers panicked and hailed an auto into which they bundled a bleeding Usha, the impacted knitting needles, and her numb mother. They instructed the driver to take the mother-daughter duo to CMC.

Usha never made it to the ward, and she never received the blood transfusion. She bled to death with her mutilated child in her perforated uterus; a sixteen-year-old lost her life that night in casualty because her desperate mother had taken her to a quack. Or had she lost her life because we had not offered her a safer option, under sterile conditions, with a trained pair of hands to terminate her mid-term pregnancy with all its complications when she had come to us first?

This is in memory of the many Ushas we saw in the early 1970s. The many Ushas who died seeking help.

One of the saddest decisions that I ever witnessed in my entire medical career was an elective abdominal hysterectomy on a mentally challenged girl who was incapable of looking after herself. Both the parents, in their late seventies and struggling with health issues of their own, knew that when the time came, they would have to depend on relatives to institutionalise her, when she would, in all probability be vulnerable and defenceless. They came seeking an abdominal hysterectomy to surgically induce menopause and prevent an unwanted pregnancy if their daughter was ever abused. The mother broke down and sobbed. She said that if we did not consider their request, there was only one option open to them. She would have to get some rat poison, mix it with their dinner, and go to bed hoping the three of them would not wake up in the morning. My heart broke to hear the despair in her voice.

To adhere to the guidelines of conducting a hysterectomy on a mentally challenged person, multiple counselling sessions were held with a psychiatrist, clinical psychologist, and a trained medical social worker. Under advisement, a written consent was obtained from her parents, and she underwent a vaginal hysterectomy with no complications. Her recovery was uneventful, and she was discharged, but not before she had endeared herself to all the staff, who watched her leave with mixed emotions.

Dermatology in London

In 1986, when Sam and I were working in Nepal, I was awarded the CIBA-GEIGY scholarship to train at the Institute of Dermatology, St John's Hospital for Diseases of the Skin,

London. The kids stayed on at Mount Hermon School in Darjeeling, and Sam joined Brompton Hospital, UK, to continue his research.

We moved into a flat in Byron Court just walking distance from the Charles Dickens Museum, which houses the author's memorabilia. Phay Ken-Lin from Singapore lived in the William Goodenough Hostel for single ladies, and Lai from Hong Kong stayed in the London House for bachelors. All three buildings faced Mecklenburgh Square, a park that led to the Underground station at Russell Square. Phay, Lai, and I would take the Underground and sometimes, William Sanchez Bothomley, a classmate from British Columbia who also lived close by, would join us. We would take the tube from Russell Square to Leicester Square, passing through Holborn and Covent Garden on the Piccadilly Line, crossing the buskers who lined the Underground.

The walk from Leicester Square to the entrance of St John's Hospital was a unique experience. St John's was a quaint old building right in the heart of the red-light area of Soho in the West End, with Chinatown, theatres, and busy pubs as immediate neighbours. Bored, busty, leggy models with pierced body parts, elaborate make-up, and false eyelashes hung out of doorways, skimpily dressed in bling and sporting snazzy stilettos, displaying their goodies while chewing gum.

Hello Love, they would pout with their come-hither looks, *Wanna come in?*

Initially, this was a playful distraction for the boys in our batch who would dawdle and trail behind, chaffing each other, much to our amusement. Soon the novelty wore off as we got serious about the course, and they did not bat an eyelid as they purposefully strode up and down Lisle Street every day. The models could have been the fire hydrants on the sidewalk for all they cared.

The Chinese takeaways in Chinatown had the succulent Peking duck hooked above steaming cauldrons of soup, bobbing up and down with a tantalising aroma wafting out, inviting us in for piping hot Dim Sums on cold winter days. The sophisticated Chinese restaurants in the West End had red oriental lanterns with knotted red tassels hanging over glass cases that showcased their illustrated menus replete with the prices. Beautiful Chinese girls in red, full-length cheongsams with high slits, gold earrings, and stilettos hovered at the ornate glass-studded wooden doors to usher in customers. The Chinese supermarkets spilt over onto the pavements, with persimmons rolling off carelessly piled heaps tripping up pedestrians as they hurried past.

The theatres, and there were enough of them in the area to call it theatre-land, had counters that opened in the afternoons, offering discounted tickets. Sometimes we would stand patiently in long serpentine queues, sacrificing our lunch break to buy tickets that suited our student budgets. We saw as much of the theatre as we possibly could and missed it sorely when we returned to India after the course. The pubs in Soho opened around 11 am. Some remained open as late-night bars to quench people's thirst in the wee hours of the morning. The gay bars had strange names and were manned by burly bouncers to remove troublemakers.

At number 5 Lisle Street, St John's Hospital, built in 1897, was an iconic old building with a quaint gabled façade, a peaked roof, and a clock tower, modelled along the lines of the early Renaissance style architecture of northern Europe. St John's faced the Swiss Centre, a popular tourist attraction that showcased all things Swiss, including the Swiss bank. The centre, a spectacular multi-storeyed tinsel mall with gourmet shops that specialised in chocolates, cheese and candy, smelled and dazzled like a Christmas tree all year round.

Dermatology inpatients were admitted to Eastern Hospital, Homerton, eight miles away. The Institute of Dermatology, a member of the British Postgraduate Medical Federation funded by the University of London, ran the dermatology course out of St John's Hospital and Eastern Hospital, mentored by Professor Malcolm Greaves and Professor Edward Wilson-Jones. The lectures were held in a little room near the clock tower right at the top of St John's Hospital for Skin Diseases. The doctors, an international bunch who had come soon after their graduation or thereabouts, were bright-eyed and bushy-tailed. Some had come after working for years in departments of dermatology in cadre posts sponsored by their governments. I had come after fifteen years of Mission service in the Himalayas with a stint at CMC for my DGO, and I was completely lost.

Initially, I felt totally out of my depth and everything zipped over my head, and I had to work extra hard to keep up as I struggled to come up for air. Sometimes, I would have panic attacks thinking that I would never pass the exams. The Ciba-Geigy Scholarship hung like a sword of Damocles over my head, along with 3-D nightmares that I was going to disgrace myself by failing the course. My batchmates, God bless them all, were extremely protective of me, and they cushioned and cossetted me and brought me up to speed, especially young Saras Sinniah, the nineteenth child of Sri Lankan parents from Malaysia. She was an absolute angel. We did everything together, including combined studies. Saras, sponsored by the government of Malaysia, had a photographic memory that stood her in good stead in a visual speciality like dermatology.

She never forgot anything that she read or saw. She took me under her wing and dragged me along with her the first few weeks of the course when I was ready to pack up and go home. Or jump off the London Bridge. Phay, Lai, and William, who had worked as dermatology registrars in their countries, grilled me all the way up and down the Piccadilly Line, and before I knew it, I was confident enough to present and discuss the cases we had to clerk. God bless them all. There was a tremendous feeling of camaraderie in the batch, and we all became good friends. Rao and Rashid were from Pakistan; Saras, Thanni, Kalyani, Gan, and Wong came from Malaysia, William from British Columbia, Maruwa from Zimbabwe, Imalingat and Kahindo from Kenya, Evelyn from the Philippines, and there were two lady doctors from Libya who lived and conversed continuously in a language and world of their own. The student from Saudi Arabia escaped to Europe after the first few classes and was never seen again.

Professor Malcolm Greaves structured an impressive course with many authors from *Rook's Textbook of Dermatology* lecturing on their specialities including Marks, Atherton, Cronin, Eady, Parish, Hawk, Bryceson, Hay, Black, Rycroft, Griffiths, Dawber, Smith, Wilson-Jones, Waters, and Camp. For the ward rounds and bedside clinics, we were taken to Eastern Hospital.

Dr Tony Bryceson, an infectious diseases expert who did tropical dermatology, had a refreshing sense of humour and punctuated his lectures with interesting anecdotes. Dracunculiasis, caused by the Guinea worm parasite, is found in Chad, Ethiopia, South Sudan, and other countries. Patients infected with it develop a blister on the leg that ruptures, with a worm emerging from the site. Dr Bryceson told us about a patient who presented at a hospital in London and gave a history of a worm that came out of his leg, looked at him, and went back inside. The doctor was clueless and sent the patient for a psychiatric evaluation. Only when the patient gave a history of travel to Africa was he referred to Tony Bryceson.

With International travel shrinking the globe, tropical diseases were no longer a rarity in the UK.

There were associations for every imaginable disease run by patients who had the disease and their caregivers, where experiences were shared to encourage others. This was a tremendous support system for old and new patients besieged with doubts and fears.

It reminded me of a story my Dad used to tell me. When a man died, he was shown heaven and hell. The rooms had people seated around a large circular dining table overflowing with food and drink. Everyone sat around the table with their arms splinted at their elbows, unable to feed themselves. Heaven and hell looked alike except for one small detail. In hell, everyone sat around unhappy and disgruntled in tamasic mode as they gazed at the gorgeous spread, ogling what they thought was inaccessible to them. *So much available but was sadly out of reach!* In heaven, they had figured out a way to fend off starvation. They fed each other with outstretched hands to reach a win-win solution. In hell they did not and would not.

Besides my training in dermatology, St John's taught me valuable lessons for life.

PART 5
Sasurean | The Samuels |

For better, for worse

Four years older than I, Sam stepped into my life in our first year in medical college and assumed charge. When I wrote and told my Mum and Dad about Sam, they had a fit. *We sent you there to study,* they chorused in anguish. The debate lasted for six years. When I threatened to stay single for the rest of my life, they finally gave in. The thought of me as a stubborn old maid on their hands must have been daunting and was probably the deciding factor for their change of heart. We got married in Christ Church on 27th November 1971.

When Evelyn Yogesvaran my bestie, the Christ Church kid I grew up with, came to help me get dressed for the wedding, she did the unthinkable. She confiscated my glasses, after telling me that I looked like an incongruous cross between Catwoman and Batwoman. She ignored my protests when I bleated that I could not even see my dreams without them. I do not know about you, but unless I see the source of sound, I cannot hear very well. I need my glasses to hear properly. So, the entire evening was a bit of a happy blur. Blind as a bat, I walked up the aisle on my Dad's arm and down the aisle on Sam's, smiling like a Cheshire cat so as not to appear rude in case someone was smiling at me.

Bishop Roland Koh was extremely taken with Sam. In his remarks from the pulpit, he said that he had never seen a bridegroom sing so well or so happily at his own wedding. My Dad, on the other hand, was not amused when Sam signed the register on the dotted line meant for the bishop. Sam said that he was so happy that we were married he would have signed all over the page!

After all the festivities were over, exhausted from shaking hands and smiling continuously, we and our stiff facial muscles crawled into my bed in the parsonage in the wee hours of the morning. No sooner had we shut our eyes than we were woken up to get ready for the 8 o'clock service in Christ Church. Rubbing his eyes incredulously, Sam muttered *Why did we bother coming home? We could have slept in the church!* After the 8 am Tamil service, my Dad took us to the 11 am Tamil service at the Epiphany Church, which he had built in the Sembawang Naval Base. When the service was over, my Dad drove us back home to the entire family—parents, uncles, aunts, and cousins—waiting to finish the leftover wedding biryani stuffed in the fridge. Somewhere between the biryani and the ice cream, Sam's father announced that he had not understood a word of the Tamil service he attended in the morning. He wanted to know if there was an English service he could attend in the evening. Before we knew it, we were *all* driven to the English evensong at St Andrew's Cathedral at 6 pm. Sam, by then, was beginning to look a bit blue around the gills and muttered under his breath to me, *I hope there are no more services anywhere else in Singapore after this!*

A week later, after we had visited every tourist spot in Singapore accompanied by the clan of uncles, aunts, and cousins in alphabetical order, we returned to India, which was in the middle of the 1971 Bangladesh war. We went to Dudgaon, now in Telangana, where Sam's father had a special service and reception to meet all Sam's family and friends. Between the Anglican canon and the Methodist pastor, they made sure that we were blessed and sanctified by every congregation they could lay their hands on after the wedding. Signed, sealed, and blessed on multiple occasions in different countries, we returned to CMC Vellore as husband and wife with the only piece of advice that my Dad gave us when we got married: *Never go to bed angry with each other,* an old-fashioned recipe to stay friends and keep a marriage together. It certainly helped us make all the adjustments we needed to start our lives together as a married couple, helping us survive all the times we wanted to strangle each other. We ended up forging a life of love and understanding that surprised even us.

We started our life together in the Men Interns' Quarters, the MIQ, at CMC in a single room on the ground floor allotted to married couples. The tiny room had a tiny bed, a tiny table, and a tiny built-in cupboard that housed all of Sam's belongings in neat and tidy piles. He was delighted that we were married and had thought far enough to extend the narrow single bed, but he was astounded that I needed to share his cupboard and table with him as he had not worked out the dynamics of marital bliss and sharing shelves in confined spaces. The extension of the bed was a temperamental plank of wood hinged down onto the side of the bed. Sometimes it behaved and stayed up on its hinges, and sometimes it did not. The person sleeping at the edge of the bed had two distinct disadvantages. Firstly, you could unceremoniously be thrown off onto the floor if the hinges decided to buckle. Secondly, if you slept on the edge, you would have to get up when the milkman banged on the door at an unearthly hour and wash the milk pan to collect the milk. Very quickly, I worked out that I was better off sleeping near the wall. Sam, good natured that he is, always ended up sleeping on the edge.

We came from similar backgrounds but grew up in different continents as ecclesiastic offspring, or pastor's kids. Though I had known Sam for six years, I rapidly learned after we were married that I really did not know the man at all. He is a lark, and I am an owl. He goes to bed early and gets up early. I go to bed late and get up late. He is a morning person who jumps out of bed bright-eyed and bushy-tailed, while I just want to bury my head in the sheets to shut out the sun. He likes sweets. I like savouries. He likes vegetables cooked beyond recognition while I like a crunch to my stir-fry. Our palates were poles apart when we set up house, but through all the years of living together in different places and cultures, we learned to adjust and accommodate. Over the years, like cake and biscuits that share a tin, bits of the cake became hard, and bits of the biscuits became soft.

Though we both are Scorpios with strong views and diametrically opposite perspectives that we cling to passionately, we talk about everything though there are some topics that have remained unresolved. We have learned to *agree to disagree* for the sake of peace and longevity. One sport we both enjoy is laughing together, often at the same jokes and with the same foolish intensity, especially at the post-mortems we hold on returning home after social gatherings. Women get their way if they cry, I am told. Not with Sam. Crying always makes Sam dig in his most obstinate heels, making me seriously toy with the idea of changing the spelling of his name to *Samule*. On the other hand, if I keep quiet for half an hour, it rattles him enough to make him give in as he absolutely hates it if I ignore him, a smart modus operandi that I have perfected over the years.

Sam the hoarder

Sam is the biggest hoarder, this side of the Suez. He hates parting with anything, which might explain why he has stuck with my craziness. In sharp contrast, I am the biggest non-collector you will ever find. I go on ruthless, exhilarating cleaning binges to declutter my life. The only problem is that if I throw things out when Sam is around, you can be sure that Sam will sit outside with a basket to collect everything and bring them back in. This ends up with no movement of throwaways. One step forward and two steps back. I soon realised that these spells of cleaning had to be done when Sam was travelling if there was to be any hope of improving the *feng shui* of our lives.

One day, when Sam was away, the Sunday school kids of St Thomas Garrison Church came around collecting odds and ends for their jumble sale. Delighted, I went on a rampage and added a pair of shoes from Sam's cupboard onto the growing pile. When Sam returned, we went to the sale and walked around aimlessly. Suddenly, Sam let out a yelp, *Susieeee!* Imagine Sam's shock and horror, when he recognised his Italian shoes lying forlornly atop a pile of faded clothes, tied together by their designer shoelaces. He was speechless.

Those are my Italian shoes, Susie he growled, as he strode towards the kids selling the jumble and said, smiling through gritted teeth, *Those are my shoes and I want them back*. You cannot fool young entrepreneurs these days, and they know a *biggie* when they see one. Uncle Sam was a great favourite with the kids at church, but they were not going to let a deal of a lifetime slip out of their teenage hands. *Uncle Sam, are these yours?* they asked, with an innocence that belied their business acumen. *You want them back, Uncle Sam? How much will you pay for them, Uncle Sam?* asked the Shadrach sisters Jwala and Jothi who were handling the jumble sale. After some relentless haggling and after an indecent sum of money had passed hands, all for a good cause I might add, the kids handed over the shoes, and I got the *Why can't you leave my things alone, Susie* lecture, ad nauseam and unabridged, all the way home in an air-conditioned car, with the windows up, when I could not escape with my famous one-liner, *There is someone at the door.*

The Samuel kids

Before we knew it, Rekha and Anish joined the family and became the pivot of our lives.

Rekha and Anish, are as different as chalk and cheese, both as kids and as adults. Born fifteen months apart, they grew up close, with Rekha protecting her baby brother and shielding him from anything or anyone who came remotely close to harming him. She used to tell the world that he was her *wonly* brother. When they were given bananas, Anish would lay them side by side to check if they were the same size. If one of them appeared longer, he would tell his sister, *Not to worry Rekha, I will fix it.* With a straight face, he would bite off the extra bit and hand her the rest of the banana that he had just bitten. For a long time, Rekha never worked out just where the extra bit of banana was going.

In Nepal

After graduating from CMC, Sam and I were posted to the Himalayan Kingdoms of Bhutan and Nepal. The kids were babies in Bhutan and could not run around the hospital campus on their own. In Nepal as preteens, they were all over the place. Rekha and Anish, *Baba* as he was called, grew up in leprosy hospitals situated in isolated locales in the Himalayas. When they returned home from school in Kathmandu, their friends were the patients in the wards and the staff who worked with us. The campus kids were much younger. John and Jenny, the Nakami kids, who were around the same age, lived with their grandparents in Kathmandu during the school term and came home only during the holidays when the four of them were inseparable as *the awesome foursome*.

Rekha and Anish acquired the nicknames *Yak and Yeti* as the guides who accompanied visitors when they came home. One of the highlights of the conducted tour was a plastering defect in one of the walls of the living room, covered by a *Thangka*, a local Bhutanese painting. They would march the visitors up to the wall, shift the *Thangka*, show them the defect and pipe up, *This is the hole in the wall that Mummy covers with a Thangka*. Innocent and deliciously honest, they would say the right thing at the wrong time, while I lived in fear and trepidation, wondering what they would say next, and to whom!

Our house was at the foot of a hill overlooking a green and lush terraced valley with a beautiful pine tree, we called *the tuning fork tree*, in the front of the kitchen. The tree trunk had bifurcated into two, just like the prongs of a tuning fork. Pine trees dropped their cones all the way up and down the paths that led to the wards and back, while the fresh smell of pine fir mingled with the almost pure and unpolluted air. Life was healthy, picturesque, and unbelievably basic. A rookie islander from Singapore, with no crash course on surviving the snow-capped mountains of the Himalayas, I shed bling and high heels to trip up and down the hillside with Rekha and Anish skipping alongside, chattering nineteen to the dozen in Nepali.

Rekha was my shadow in the wards, the labour room, and the theatre. She would follow me everywhere, happy just to be with me. When we operated, she would sit on the window ledge reading a book. Anish did not like the sight or smell of blood. He practically lived in the carpenter's shed, helping to repair patient trolleys and wheels. If not there, he would be in the garage playing with the drivers behind the wheel of the stationary hospital jeep. The maintenance staff loved him as much as he did them. Anish and Rekha roamed up and down the hill, playing with patients and staff, totally oblivious to the stigma attached to a leprosy hospital. An aunt who came to spend a holiday with us was aghast. Desperately concerned and in utter disbelief, she asked me *Are you sure about all this leprosy stuff?*

The British Primary School, Kathmandu

Every morning the kids and Tularam the postman would leave on a bumpy mud road for the British Primary School in Kathmandu with Sathya, their favourite school driver at the wheel of the Land Rover. Sathya was a kind and gentle human being who loved our kids and looked after them as if they were his own. If they were hungry on their way back from school, he would stop at Ram Bhandar, the local tea shop and buy them piping hot samosas, a savoury puff with a potato filling. If we were busy at the hospital when they came home from school, Sathya would warm the food on the kitchen table and feed them. We never worried about the welfare or safety of our kids as long as they were with the hospital staff who looked after them like their own.

Their *Show and Tell* sessions at school had their teachers in splits. Rekha's teacher Anne Scholey, a dear friend, would ring up to read out Rekha's nuggets, punctuated with helpless giggles.

> *Mummy and Daddy had a fight. Daddy said he's leaving and Mummy asked who will have you?*
> *Mummy's uncle came to visit us and he never brought us any presents.*
> *My Mummy cut off a patient's leg today*
> *When I get bigger and Mummy gets smaller...I will...*

do this…or that…or the other.
Uncle xxxx came for a holiday and he forgot to close the door when he was having a bath.
Mummy found all the food we threw out of the window.
My Daddy refuses to write his will.
My Mummy mauled a bear in Bhutan.
My Daddy came home yesterday after searching for patients in the mountains. Mummy made him take off all his clothes outside because he had leeches in his pants.

Our home was a popular sleepover destination for their school friends. Anandaban Hospital, built in a clearing in a pine forest, had no fences or gates. No roads to cross. No crazy traffic. No horns.

There were trees to climb, slopes to roll down, and you could kick a ball for as far as your eye could see without any fear of breaking glass. For kids growing up in Kathmandu, Anandaban was as close to heaven as they got. The kids who tumbled out of the Land Rover in various stages of disarray looked like next-gen delegates arriving for a United Nations conference. They attended the British Primary while their parents, expats from all over the world, worked on a foreign posting in Nepal. When they came home after playing and rolling over field and slope, they would have a bath, change into their pyjamas, and come hurtling down the steps to jostle around our kitchen table, ravenously hungry. Piping hot puffed up *poori*s rolled up and eaten with jam or sugar was a popular treat, especially with young Ben Bury, who sat at the table with sugar all over his face and ginger hair, happily mouthing, *boori*s, *boori*s. There was no telling what adventures the *poori*s would have en route to being eaten. Some transformed into missiles to be hurled at others during the airstrikes they staged around the crowded kitchen table. When we ran out of *pooris*, we would knead fresh dough and roll it out on the kitchen top to cut fresh batches, a task they all enjoyed helping in with gay abandon as flour, dough cutter, and rolling pin flew all over the kitchen, almost like a craft class gone awry.

Mount Hermon School

Soon we had to make the painful decision of sending the kids away to boarding school. Mount Hermon in Darjeeling, run by Rev. John Johnston and his wife, Val, came highly recommended as the natural choice. When we entered the headmaster's office, we thought Hollywood's Robert Redford was shooting his next film in the school. Rev. Johnston had the same good looks, shy smile, and the brightest blue eyes I had ever seen. Eyes that twinkled at you with infinite kindness and understanding. He took us around after the formalities of admission were over, and we got to see him interact with the little ones who were in the playground for a break. When they saw him, they all ran to him spontaneously, shouting and scrambling for his attention. Many flung themselves at him as he stopped to ruffle their hair, straighten a tie, or give them a hug. One thing was abundantly clear, he seemed to know each child by name and it was obvious that they all loved him.

Sam used to accompany them to Darjeeling to drop them off at school. Rekha's little chin would quiver, and she would wipe her tears and Sam's tears with her little hand and say, *Daddy don't cry, please don't cry.* Anish used to cling to Sam's shirt, bury his crumpled little face in Sam's tummy, and sob, *Daddy, don't go. Daddy, please don't go.* It used to break Sam's heart, and he used to blubber so much that the Johnstons christened him

Waterworks. The kids, I am told, would be fine within the hour as they were taken out to play and were distracted by the teachers and wardens. Sam, on the other hand, stricken by remorse, would cry all the way home. Sam's Dad, Rev. NS Mathew, was a Nirmal missionary and a minister of the Methodist church in the Medak Diocese and Sam's Mum, Alice, was a teacher. Since they worked in transferrable postings to remote villages in Andhra Pradesh, they too had to make the painful decision of putting their three sons, Sam, John, and Prem in the Wesley Boys School and Boarding in Secunderabad.

Sam was just six years old when he joined the boarding. When his Dad dropped him off at school, father and son used to cry. Sam used to clutch the front of his Dad's cassock and cry, *Daddy, don't go, Daddy, please don't go*. Sam made a promise to himself that he would never send his kids to a boarding school. A promise he sadly could not keep.

Val and John were ever so kind during their protracted and heart-breaking farewells. Their reassuring wave and smile was the last memory Sam always took with him as he drove back to Kathmandu. We were comforted knowing that our kids, though far from us, were in the care of the Johnstons.

When the kids went away to boarding school, we threw ourselves completely into our work.

The ache of missing Rekha and Anish was almost physical, like a hole in my heart. I agree that they were just kids, but they were my faithful companions on the snow-capped mountains. I missed them terribly, especially when I went home after work. Perhaps that's why my *Velliammachy* had 19 kids - she made sure that she never had an empty nest !

Fresh off the boat

The best years of my life as a Mum, were spent in the Pilgrim Lodge, the Leprosy Mission House in Kew Gardens, London. The kids were delightful companions in a land where every day was an adventure. We were so poor, we had no wheels to take them great distances on road trips. We just took them to the magnificent Kew Gardens through one of its different gates, and the kids thought it was a new venue every time. They would roll on the grass and when the pond was not frozen, feed the ducks with the stale bread they had saved at home. An outgoing pair of siblings, they would make friends easily. On my birthday, Rekha and Anish broke free and ran down the pavement of Ennerdale Road, which Anish pronounced as *Ennerdilady*, informing complete strangers that it was my birthday. *It's my Mummy's birthday today,* they chimed in unison, *and she is thirty-two years old!*

One morning we tripped over to watch the Changing of the Guard at Buckingham Palace. As we could not see anything, we slipped under the cordon and got to see everything ringside, thanks to the kind folks at the venue. I would take the kids to museums, art galleries, flea markets, and all the places I wanted to go and they skipped along happily as Sam, who was working on his PhD, left home before the sun came up and walked in only after the 10 o'clock news.

Young Anish was a regular at the ER of the local hospital where the nurses would exclaim, *Well, well, well, look who's back?* One winter, he had new mittens on for school when he climbed up the climbing frame. When I walked through the gate, he became so excited he shouted, *Look Mummy look!* One minute he was up there and the next minute he was on the cemented floor, several feet below the bar he was swinging on, with his arm hanging by his side at a sinister angle. The school, fearing an impending lawsuit that never happened, turned offensive in their defence and scolded me for coming late. Another occasion I remember clearly was a Sunday morning when we were getting ready to go to St Luke's church around the corner, when Anish ran and crashed into a glass cupboard at the end of the room. What I saw when I looked turned my blood into ice. His head had gone through the glass, shattering it, leaving a spiky piece of glass pointing upwards, ready to pierce his neck if he moved. I froze in horror. When I tried to call out to Sam, no words came out of my mouth. Rekha had meanwhile run into the study and returned with Sam, who fortunately was home on a Sunday. With great presence of mind and extremely steady hands, Sam extricated Anish from the broken glass cupboard with Rekha navigating the entire operation. I just watched in rigor mortis.

Sam babysits Chicken Licken

When I joined the Margaret Pyke Family Planning Clinic in London, I met Dr Cooper, the kindly Parsi lady who ran the clinic. Extremely sympathetic, she worked me into their flexible hours, allotting me sessions when the kids were in school. Walking past the shops around Oxford Circus, window shopping and ogling all the way made Sam wonder if I had spent the day's income even before I reached the clinic! Since the NHS in the early seventies offered a fully comprehensive contraceptive service free of cost with open access, the footfall at the clinic was an interesting mix of the very young and the old. The youngest patient I saw was all of ten years when she became pregnant while on contraceptives. Models and professional dancers would chalk up every ounce they gained on the pill and starve themselves to lose it all. Since I worked in a sari, the Indians, Bangladeshis and Pakistanis would remove their charts from my pile. I believe I reminded them of their

Mums and aunts and their consults would have been too close to home!

Once a week on Wednesdays, I had a late-night session at MPC when Sam would babysit the kids. Rekha and Anish would be waiting for me on the steps leading upstairs when I let myself in with a *Shoosh Mummy, we've just managed to get Daddy to sleep!* Sure enough, when we entered their bedroom Sam would be fast asleep on the armchair next to their bunk beds with Ladybird's *Chicken Licken* open on his chest. He would have supervised their baths, made them an omelette dinner and put them down reading *Chicken Licken*. When he tried desperately to miss the pages of repeats of *Chicken Licken, Henny Penny, Cocky Locky* etc, the kids always caught him out and made him go back. To the kids' delight, after several failed attempts of skipping pages, he always dropped off exhausted!

Julia Welchman

I would never have survived England if Julia Welchman and Helene Alexander King, mothers with kids at the same school, had not picked me up from the school gate. The Welchmans, Julia, Malcolm, Anthea and Jocelyn kept open house with Julia as *Yellow Pages* to the young expat Mums she rescued from the school gate. She was our go-to person when we needed help with absolutely anything. When I first saw Julia, she was standing in the middle of the road shaking her fist at a truck driver speeding down the school road.

Absolutely fearless, she would take on anyone or anything that threatened to disturb the peace of the Kew community. Altruistic to a fault, Julia had perfected a wonderful community support system to help young Mums living overseas for the first time. The Welchman home was a treasure trove of useful stuff that they could borrow, free of cost, until they got their own.

There were pots and pans, prams, cycles, musical instruments, clothes to fit all ages, fancy dress costumes and woollies—you name it, Julia had it! When we returned what we borrowed, we made sure that we topped it up with a little extra something to help another new Mum on the block, our way of paying back and sustaining Julia's project.

Helene Alexander King
Helene drove her kids to school in a yellow SUV. Hers was the only family who was later than the Samuels; she would always stop and let us crawl into the back. After we dropped the kids off, she would drive me around and we would talk. Helene was my personal tutor, the one who broke me in, showed me the ropes, and settled me into life in England. Though I was so painfully naïve and *fresh off the boat,* Helene never ever scoffed. She took me everywhere and taught me everything I needed to know. In the departmental stores and grocery stores, we would walk around the counters watching the demos. She gave me the most precious gift of all: her time and counsel. I remember us visiting Phyllis, a friend from church who had moved into a retirement home in Kew. There was an unusual flurry of activity as they were getting ready for a wedding in the afternoon. Two of their residents, a ninety-five-year-old and a ninety-three-year-old were tying the knot before moving into their own pad with double bed, diapers and all. The elderly did not curl up waiting to die; they lived in hope and love, thanking God for every extra day they were given! They never lost their *joie de vivre!*

Helene's family was singularly inclusive with friends all over the world. Why their kids, Charlie, Lucy and Tom, my godson, were all given an international bunch of godparents including Bishop Desmond Tutu who was their parish priest in Golders Green.

Rekha and the goat

Rekha started her driving lessons in the Defence Colony grounds in Chennai, an open space where the villagers let their livestock graze. It was not uncommon to see red L-plates weaving between livestock. One morning, Rekha came back from the class a little shaken. She said that they had had a near miss with a goat on the field, but luckily the goat had run off unscathed. Neither of us gave the incident another thought when we left in a little while, she for college and I for the clinic.

Our gate was always kept locked as the dogs would run out given half a chance. When they heard the car horn, all four dogs would rush out and jump at the locked gate, barking wildly. They made such a ruckus that I am sure that our neighbours, the Chadhas next door, would have complained bitterly, or moved, had they not been passionate dog lovers themselves, with half a dozen dogs in their compound at any point of time. Clayton, our cook, would come to the gate in his colourful Bermuda shorts and T-shirt to shoo all the dogs behind the wicker gate in front of the garage and close it carefully before he opened the main gate to let the car in. This could take from ten to fifteen minutes, depending on how frisky and excited the dogs were to see us and on how sober Clayton was. This was all the time it would take Anish, who would have come back from school by then, to hang out of his window and give me a blow-by-blow account of all of that had happened while I was away. *Mummy, you will never guess what happened today,* he would start in his best conspiratorial voice, and then proceed to tell me exactly what had happened not missing any gory detail. I was always well informed before I entered the home. I knew exactly who had done what, to whom, when, and where.

When Rekha and I returned that evening, I noticed that Anish was more excited than usual and bursting with news.

Rekha, do you know what you did? You killed a goat! He kept repeating as he jumped up and down. Rekha paled in fright, and looked as if she was going to burst into tears. Parking the car, we ran in fearfully as Anish greeted us with an elaborate *show and tell* while he pranced around with his audio-visual embellishments. Sam was at home when a belligerent crowd arrived half an hour after Rekha and I had left home demanding money for the goat they claimed Rekha had killed. He listened very carefully and made suitable noises at all the right places.

He promised to pay up when they brought him the dead goat. In his mind's eye, we were sitting down to mutton biryani for dinner. They were flummoxed as there was no goat to produce in exchange for the money. They conferred among themselves and left threatening to come back with the goat. They did not return, and Sam thought that he had seen the last of them, when at 4 pm a thinner, more subdued crowd arrived at the gate with the head of a goat. It was a dry specimen with no trace of blood, looking suspiciously like the dismembered head of a goat that usually hangs on display at a butcher's shop after a goat is slaughtered for meat. Sam stood his ground as the group hemmed and hawed and finally left shuffling sheepishly without any money passing hands. Though Rekha did finish her driving course and passed her driving test, we could never pass a goat without Anish teasing her mercilessly as only a brother can. *Look Rekha...Goat... Look Rekha look... Goatie... Goatie... Look Rekha, look...*

Shrek One & Shrek Two
Being the only child of elderly parents left me severely handicapped as an adult. One of the skills I lacked was swimming. I was never allowed swimming lessons in case I drowned, just as I was never allowed to learn cycling or driving.

My Mum and Dad worried that I would either kill myself or worse, kill an unsuspecting pedestrian. One day, many years later, watching my grandkids Ashish and Rohan, in the pool, it struck me that I was so wrong to think that I did not know how to swim. Of course, I knew how to swim! I was swimming in utero even before I walked. I just needed to refresh what I already knew.

When I shared my earth-shattering discovery with Sam, he agreed to come for swimming lessons. Sam and I, both in our sixties, enrolled at a swimming camp in Chennai. These camps are designed primarily for schoolchildren during the summer holidays. The average age of the children at that particular camp was nine, which made us instantly prehistoric. We did not care. We were just desperate to learn swimming. We ran the idea by Rekha and Anish, both ace swimmers. I had insisted that they learn swimming, cycling, and driving early in life so that they would not struggle in their adult years. They were extremely encouraging and cheered us on. *Mummy, when you make soup, the fat floats on top, right?* Anish said. *So, don't worry, you will never drown!* he said, to reassure me, I think.

When we arrived at the pool, we found a bunch of exuberant kids in swimsuits around a young man who squinted at us with an amused expression as he watched the two elderly eager beavers join the line of squealing children. This was the most important man in our lives for the next eight weeks: our swimming instructor, *Saravanan Sir*. Sending up a quick prayer, we placed our lives in his hands. When we met the lady at the desk for our swimsuits, she never measured us for size. She merely looked us up and down, handed us our packets, and directed us to the slippery changing rooms that reeked of chlorine. My swimsuit was a deep purple spandex one-size-fits-all. I could not believe my eyes when I held it against me and looked in the mirror on the wall. It looked like a leotard with a tutu stitched around the hips. Even if it did nothing else, it would cover me from my wrists to my knees. Then I did a vigorous *Naagin* snake dance , with much optimistic pulling and pushing of obstinate body parts to coax them into places they really did not want to go to or could not possibly fit into. This took almost thirty minutes.

In far better shape than I was, Sam had no trouble getting into his swimming trunks. Stuffing his clothes into his swim bag, he kept watching the swivel door of the ladies' changing room, waiting for me to emerge. Confused when he did not see me come out, he wondered if I had beaten him to the pool. When he went around to the pool, he did not find me there either. Half an hour later, he became a little restless and sent the attendant to check if I had slipped or passed out on the floor. Or fled. Sheepishly, I emerged anxious minutes later and walked with mincing steps to the shower at the edge of the pool, with Sam following me, not daring to laugh. *Don't you dare say a word Sama,* I hissed as I showered and lowered myself gingerly into the cold water. The frilly tutu bit broke the ice. It was of no use to man or beast, and it certainly was of no use to me. As soon as I got into the water, it floated up like a damp equator around my midriff, reducing me, a visibly relieved Sam, the kids in the pool, and the curious spectators around the pool to ripples of hysterical laughter.

A few minutes later, Anish came to see how we were doing. When he saw his elderly parents floundering like a pair of drowning ducks among a bunch of noisy kids splashing in the pool, he laughed so much and so hard he almost fell into the pool. *Good grief!* he gasped, coming up for air, *You look like Shrek One and Shrek Two!* Undeterred, Sam and I persisted with the classes and eventually learned to swim rather well. With time, the ridiculous spandex became a whimsical memory we traded for a practical swim dress that covered the essentials and did not float up with a mind of its own.

Sasurean

Sasurean, an acronym for the homes that Sam, Susie, Rekha, and Anish lived in all the corners of the world, has always been shared by an odd assortment of human beings and others. Anish's love for animals surfaced early in life and his love of fish is legendary.

We had fish in all shapes and colours swimming in tanks all over the house. Tanks that leaked, tanks that creaked, tanks that overflowed, and tanks that did not. At one stage, when we lived at 208 Defence Colony, we had four dogs of different breeds; two man-eating baby piranhas in a cement tank in the garden; a golden arowana that swam alone in a six-foot tank in the front veranda; an Oscar and an assorted school of fish swimming in a tank in the dining room; a checkered keelback snake that roamed the house when it wasn't in Anish's pocket; for a short while, Dodi, a baby bull tied to the mango tree in the centre of our backyard; and a blur of white lovebirds that pelted poop indiscriminately on the back veranda.

On the day Anish came home with the snake, it came out of his shirt pocket, crawled around his neck, and wriggled back into his pocket. I looked on in horror while Baba looked at his performing reptile with pride, *Look Mummy…Look!* The bored snake had us panicking when it decided to leave the confines of Anish's front pocket. All hell broke loose when Anish ran down the steps yelling, *The snake has gone! The snake has gone!* We dropped everything we were doing and searched high and low for something we really did not want to find. It took us all day to find Mr Snake curled comfortably at the altar we had near the entrance.

Another day he came home with a baby bull he christened Dodi. When we tried to persuade him to leave Dodi on our acre on the East Coast Road with an underworked and overpaid caretaker to look after him, he refused. Dodi was tied to the mango tree in the centre of our cemented backyard, sharing space with our four dogs: Snoopy, Tootsie, Tiny, and Pappoo. If you looked out of our window, you would see the baby bull and four K9s living in peace and harmony under the shade of the spreading mango tree. That was fine during the dry months in Chennai. When it started raining one night, the dogs ran for shelter, without a backward glance at their differently hoofed friend. Poor Dodi could not run as he was tied to the mango tree.

Anish woke up to thunder and lightning and came charging into our room yelling, *Mummy, wake up, wake up. We have to get Dodi out of the rain. Mummy, wake up.* I leapt out of bed and followed him down the stairs. We opened the back door, ran out, and untied Dodi, who was shivering in the rain. Clutching him close, Anish ran and placed him on the tiled back veranda. Four wet hooves on a smooth tiled surface can only go one way. Dodi slipped and slithered all over the place as did Anish, who was also drenched. Not to be left out, I jumped into the fray and the three of us glissaded in gay abandon over the green tiles of the balcony. Finally, we managed to grip the grill and hoist ourselves up.

Speechless, I watched Anish run into the house and reappear with the new spare mattress from the guest room. He laid it down on the floor and carried Dodi to dry cotton. Relieved, Dodi decided to relieve himself and rained even sized, black pellets all over the mattress. Not to be left out, the K9s came in from the rain and jumped onto the mattress, pellets and all, shaking themselves furiously from side to side, as they rolled on the mattress in gay abandon to dry their rain-drenched coats. Meanwhile, the white lovebirds—who, after being rudely awakened, were watching the free entertainment from the safety of their dry cages—perched in single file and protested in shrill, discordant notes of fear. The sets of Anish's opera, *the menagerie,* were now slipping from the gross to the ridiculous.

In the morning, Anish, without a word, packed Dodi into the back of his Gypsy and drove him to the acre on the ECR.

Our K9s

Bouncy, the first dog we ever loved and lost was a beautiful Lhasa Apso who was my shadow when we were at the Gidakom Hospital in Bhutan until she was kidnapped one afternoon and plucked cruelly out of our lives. When Bouncy went missing, I never thought I could or would love another dog enough to go through the heartache of losing it again. I was so wrong.

Anish made a career of bringing puppies home. When he brought them home, he would look as woebegone as the K9. *You will never see him Mummy. You will never hear him, I promise; I will walk the dog, I will feed the dog, I will bathe the dog... just watch... Please Mummy... Promise Mummy... Please Mummy,* he would aver. Wild promises on his part and wishful thinking on mine. Of course, I knew that none of this would happen and that I would be left holding the puppy, literally. Being a sucker for puppy love, I could never say *No*.

Tiny and Pappoo, Lhasa Apso siblings, joined our family when we worked in the Anandaban Hospital in Nepal. When Rekha and Anish were at boarding school in Darjeeling, they would address their childish scrawls to Daddy-Sam, Choochie-Mummy, Tiny Samuel, and Pappoo Samuel because they considered Pappoo and Tiny family, their siblings who walked on all fours.

Pappoo, the girl, lived with us in Nepal, and Tiny, the boy, with my Mum and Dad in Chennai until we moved to Chennai when they were reunited. Seeing their joyous reunion, I had to sit them down and explain that they were siblings. *Don't ever forget that you are brother and sister*, I said in a firm voice emphasising the *brother and sister* bit.

Unfortunately, it fell on deaf ears. They indulged in romantic interludes when they would be off food and drink and mope around the house like a pair of lovesick teenagers. As Pappoo was spayed, we did not inherit an incestuous bunch of Lhasa Apsos. Like all small breeds, they lived to love us for a long time.

Devoted to me, Pappoo was the sweetest little puppy I have ever known. She knew every little nuance of my mood. She knew if I was sad. She knew if I was happy. She knew if I was angry. She just knew me.

When I came home, she would lift her little head and puppy-talk to me, asking me where I had gone and why I was so late coming back. She followed me everywhere, even waiting outside the bathroom with her nose pressed against the door until I came out and tripped over her. She never paid much attention to visitors, but if she growled at someone, we stopped in our tracks and took a second look. She and Tiny had a sixth sense to suss people out, and surprisingly, their judgment was never wrong.

Pappoo died of mammary tumours at the age of eighteen. When I took her to the Madras Veterinary Hospital, I knew the diagnosis before they told me. It was malignant, something I did not want to hear, as I was hoping against hope that my gut feeling was wrong. When they told me that she would not live more than a few weeks, I broke down and howled like a wounded animal in front of the hospital staff. The late Prof

Archibald David managed to calm me down eventually and sent us home.

Pappoo lived for a few weeks after that fateful visit. I was sleeping with her on the floor in the bedroom when she passed on. I must have dozed off when she moved closer to me and nudged me awake with a feeble paw. I shot up straight and saw her looking at me with infinite sadness in her eyes as she inched closer to me. I gathered her in my arms, held her close, and watched helplessly as she slipped away from me after eighteen glorious years together. Tiny, who was also in the bedroom, walked up, gave her a couple of perfunctory sniffs, and went off silently to curl up under the bed.

I was bereft when Pappoo left me. I fell to pieces even as Tiny, coping better than I was, comforted me. I could not make myself get off the sofa for days, and I paid no heed when the vendors cycled around the colony shouting out their wares. The fishmonger was a smart entrepreneur. He knew that he needed an infallible business strategy to get me out of the grieving mode for his sales to recover. One day, he arrived with a wiggly white powder puff instead of the assortment of seafood he usually carried in the basket at the back of his bicycle. I refused to take a look. The powder puff whimpered, and I looked. He then held the powder puff up and begged me to touch it. I refused. In a desperate attempt, he threw an ace sales pitch. He pretended to drop the powder puff onto the floor right under my nose. Instinctively, I jumped to the rescue and before I knew it, the powder puff—Pappoo the Pomeranian—was in my arms and in my heart. Tiny, who was lying under the bed, suddenly came alive and walked up to sniff her all over with a few licks and barks of approval. Pappoo the Pomeranian was exactly what the doctor had ordered for Tiny. With the young and frisky puppy around him, the eighteen-year-old listless Lhasa Apso morphed into a rejuvenated K9 who lived four more years to twenty-two dog years, which is equivalent to a hundred and fifty-four human years. I never forgot the comfort that Pappoo the Pomeranian was to me when I was grieving. Many years later, when my secretary, Mr Bala, and his wife Luieza were grieving and inconsolable, I loaned Pappoo to them for a while, to live with them and to mop up their tears. They were delighted to have Pappoo and looked after her like a baby. Unfortunately, she missed us terribly. One morning, when Mr Bala was getting ready for his bath, Pappoo darted out of their top floor flat in Choolaimedu and ran down onto the road and began weaving through the chaotic traffic. Mr Bala, dressed only in a towel, ran and caught up with her. When he brought her home to us, Pappoo was limp and exhausted after her aborted escape bid and slept under our bed for days without moving.

Snoopy, our Dalmatian, believed that I was his mother. I was his go-to person when he was hungry, scared, or sleepy. When firecrackers exploded non-stop during the many Indian festivals, he crawled under the bed whimpering pathetically or jumped into my lap if I was anywhere within leap. Though he was the largest of the pack, he was undisputedly the baby of the bunch and the most disobedient of the lot. If we said sit, he stood up and wagged his tail. If we pulled his leash to the left, he pulled to the right. His mind seemed to process orders only inversely.

When we moved to the farmhouse in Chennai, we found him a trainer from the local village, Uthandi: a policeman who had trained many police dogs. The trainer never needed to ring the bell to announce his arrival. We knew he was at the gate when Snoopy dashed in and buried his head in my sari petticoat. Looking down, I would see a black-and-white spotted sausage with a heaving chest, thumping its tail on the floor. He thought that if he buried his face, the rest of him was invisible. Cajoling him, I would drag him out to the garden when he would give me a betrayed expression with all shades of a *How could you?*

Snoopy the Dalmatian fell for Tiny the beautiful brown Labrador and sired a litter of puppies with a pedigree of their own. When she went into labour, I separated her from her curious companions and took her up to the terrace for the whelping. Tiny relying completely on her maternal instincts was absolutely marvellous for a first-time Mum. When Tiny was done, I was crying. Completely bowled over by the wonder of the whelping process I had just witnessed, my first actually. I was overwhelmed by her absolute trust in me. She lay there exhausted with her head in my lap and looked up at me with her beautiful green eyes as I sat next to her and stroked her brown coat. Truly an epiphany moment if ever there was one. Eventually, an exhausted Tiny-the-Lab climbed into the whelping box and lay there passively, even as the little wiggly pink sausages found their way instinctively to nestle close to her and feel their way to suckle.

What on earth would you call a cross between a Dalmatian and a Labrador? *Dalradors? Labmatians?* A good-looking bunch of puppies, they had no problem finding loving homes. They were all chocolate with a splash of white on the chest and paws, looking like liveried butlers wearing a waistcoat, socks, and mittens. Even the runt was good-looking, smaller but just as good-looking. Not one of them had spots or looked like Snoopy. Tiny the Lab was the only girl who carried Snoopy's pups. Tootsie was spayed, and Pappoo always snapped at Snoopy when he went sniffing. She took her virginity very seriously.

There was no trouble in paradise when Snoopy was the undisputed King of the Samuel K9-dom. Skirmishes happened only when he overlapped with the ageing male Lhasa Apso Tiny and later with the male boxer Tyson. Tiny thought *he* was the alpha dog and size did not matter. Snoopy, still a puppy, would rush out to play with Tiny, thinking it was a game. An incensed Tiny, though several sizes smaller than Snoopy, would jump up to attack him from below and end up getting his teeth caught in the loose folds of skin on Snoopy's lower jaw. The sight of Tiny hanging suspended from Snoopy's lower jaw, flailing his limbs in mid-air even as Snoopy desperately tried to shake him off, would have been quite comic had it not been for Tiny's piteous plight. Eventually, someone would unhook Tiny and put him out of his misery, though he never learned his lesson and always went for more.

Another treasure that Anish brought home was Tootsie, a cross between a Doberman and a German shepherd. A sleek black beauty with a shiny coat and a docked tail, she was a gift from Uncle Gopi. Her fierce demeanour belied the sweet and loving nature she reserved for the family. One deep throated growl from Tootsie was enough to frighten any trespasser away. Our K9s loved their vet Dr Sumeetha Antonysamy. The minute she entered the gate, they would rush to crowd her, knocking her petite frame to the ground, clamouring for her attention. After an enthusiastic welcome, they would settle down around her while she examined each one of them in great detail, whispering sweet nothings in their ears, all of which they seemed to understand perfectly.

Our K9s formed a protective band around us with a love bordering on devotion, as they kept us safe in all the lonely and isolated places we lived in.

The grand-peas

Parenting does not come with a manual, and kids do not come with a user guide. As parents, we are flawed despite all our best intentions simply because we are inexperienced humans in unfamiliar roles. Being a parent makes sense to them and to us, when we see our kids raise their kids in the sitcoms of their generation.

I delivered both my grandsons, Ashish and Rohan in diametrically opposed circumstances. Ashish was born in Shimla in 2001 under suboptimal conditions: no equipped operation theatre, no blood bank, no oxygen, and no attending paediatrician.

Rohan was born four years later in Chennai in a state-of-the-art corporate hospital with a theatre on alert; blood cross-matched; and a friend, Benny Benjamin, the neonatologist in attendance. Ashish unlocked a cascade of emotions that I did not know lived inside my heart when he was born. He taught me how to be a grandmother, a role I had worked on by the time Rohan arrived. Ashish and Rohan, four years and poles apart, fit snugly into the chambers of my heart and keep me on my toes with all the adventures they share with me.

One evening, we were sitting around after dinner when a debate found me on the side of the grand-peas with their parents Anish and Vidhu squarely on the opposite side. Anish could not believe that I would side with the grand-peas over something I may not have approved of when he was growing up. Unable to control himself, he burst out, *Ashish, this is not the lady I grew up with. This is some old lady who is trying to get into heaven!* He was absolutely right. I turned soft after the arrival of the grand-peas. What had appeared to be completely non-negotiable when our kids were growing up really did not seem so inflexible with the grandkids. The grand-peas could get their way with me in most things. These changes did not go unnoticed by their father who protested vociferously whenever he could.

As babies, the grandkids followed me around chattering like an appreciative audience. During my baking expeditions, they fought over who could lick the mixing bowl and spoon of anything remotely chocolatey, sharing them only when they brought their friends over for sleepovers to *Grandma's House*. Bedtimes were special when we got to cuddle and read all the timeless tales our kids had devoured. *Chicken Licken, Red Riding Hood, The Three Billy Goats Gruff, The Three Little Pigs*, and many from the newer Dr Seuss series, including *Green Eggs and Ham*. The years zipped past with astonishing speed, and soon they were athletic young men with funky hairstyles, spending hours at the gym. Young men who conversed as young adults to bring me up to speed with their lingo, music, men, matters, and girls. Sam and I do share a special bond with our grand-peas. Though grandparenting too comes without a manual, it is not difficult.

There are no failures in grandparenting as there are in parenting. The difference between parenting and grandparenting lies in our responses, which improve with age and experience. Primarily because we realise that it is okay to lose a battle to win a war!

PART 6

Bhutan | Nepal

The sadness in their eyes

Sam introduced me to leprosy, Dr Victor Preetam Das and The Leprosy Mission. Sam's interest in leprosy started during his BSc days, when he was an undergraduate in MCC – the Madras Christian College, Tambaram from 1961-1964. Passionately involved with the SCM – the Student Christian Movement of the College, he was an enthusiastic volunteer at the Pammal Leprosy Clinic run by the SCM. Rolling up his sleeves, he spent time with the leprosy patients dressing their ulcers. When he represented the SCM Pammal Leprosy Clinic at the All India Leprosy conference in Hyderabad in January 1963 he met Dr VP Das, the Secretary for South East Asia of the Leprosy Mission – a chance meeting that changed his whole life. Dr Das, extremely impressed with young Sam, told him that if he ever wanted to become a doctor, the Leprosy Mission would be extremely happy to sponsor his studies to CMC, the Christian Medical College, Vellore. Sam joined CMC in 1964 after he completed his BSc, sponsored by the Leprosy Mission, with a service commitment of five years in return for the sponsorship.

Sam and I joined the Leprosy Mission in 1971 as young medical graduates. The SPG, the Society for the Propagation of the Gospel to Foreign and Heathen Lands in Singapore had sponsored my medical studies at CMC with a service commitment to serve a SPG Hospital in Singapore. Since the SPG had no hospitals left in Singapore when I finished, my bond was transferred to the Leprosy Mission, which meant that Sam and I could complete our bonds together in half the time.

In the early 1970s, sharing experiences between the two hemispheres, the East and the West, was lopsided. One had patients, the other had resources, and both fumbled for knowledge in an era when communication was slow and just another difficult word to spell. To many, leprosy still conjured up visions of tattered rags huddled in heaps at roadsides that occasionally shuffled to beg. Others thought of leprosy patients as people who were interred in charitable institutions far from civilization. Either way they were dismissed as discards of the human race, deleted by their family and loved ones.

For several years, we worked in leprosy hospitals in India, Bhutan, Nepal and for a brief period in Kenya. As part of my training, I visited several hospitals the world over including the Leonard Wood Memorial Centre for Leprosy Research in Cebu, the Philippines, and the National Leprosarium in Carville, Louisiana, US. The hospitals were different, as were the medical facilities. In some leprosy hospitals overseas, the patients seemed to have a better quality of life. They lived in relatively luxurious wards and rooms, slept on softer beds, ate better food, and had access to a wider range of recreational activities and entertainment.

They enjoyed better creature comforts than our patients did. In Carville, some patients even had private yachts and limousines parked around the hospital. Medical facilities were certainly state-of-the art when funding was not a problem. However, no matter where the patients lived, whether in the US, Asia, Africa, or anywhere in the world, one thing was constant: the sad, betrayed, sometimes sightless, eyes of the patients we met. When they looked up to greet you, their eyes had a sad resignation that spoke volumes, reflecting the pain and hopelessness they felt while living out a disease that crippled them, physically and socially. Reconstructive surgery, facelifts, prosthetic limbs, restoration of function, and loving acceptance certainly gave them a new lease of life. However, the sadness in their eyes never went away.

Leprosy, aka *Hansen's disease*, is a chronic infectious disease caused by *Mycobacterium leprae*, a bacillus that resembles *Mycobacterium tuberculosis*. It affects nerves and causes distinctive skin lesions and tell-tale deformities. The tubercle bacillus has been grown in the lab in vitro and studied to develop a vaccine to prevent its spread. *M. leprae*, unfortunately, has not been grown in the lab and therefore, has not been studied well enough for a vaccine to be developed. *M. leprae* can be grown only in vivo - in animal models like the nine-banded armadillo, nude mice, and the chimpanzee.

Reconstructive Surgery

The nerves of the human upper and lower limbs have a sensory component and a motor component. When leprosy affects the motor part of a nerve, the muscles supplied by that nerve are paralysed. When it affects the sensory part of the nerve, sensation over the area of skin it supplies is lost, causing anaesthetic patches. Sensation is as crucial as it is protective. Sensation causes pain, making us stop, move away, rest and heal. When sensation is lost, injuries are discovered late, and sometimes only after infection sets in.

Every joint has two sets of muscles that pull in opposite directions: one set of muscles that flexes the joint and another that extends it. If the flexors are paralysed, the extensors act unopposed and vice versa. In leprosy, the flexors of the fingers are paralysed, and the extensors contract excessively, causing the characteristic *claw hand deformity*. In a claw hand, the palm is turned inside out. When patients try to pick up anything, they are actually pushing it away from them. This interferes with all the fine movements of the hand, including grasp and grip. If the thumb is involved simultaneously, the hand resembles that of an ape, causing *the simian hand deformity* when the thumb is unable to move forward to pinch or grasp.

Leprosy patients develop a *foot drop deformity* when the flexor muscles of the foot are paralysed and the extensors contract unopposed. When patients put their foot forward to take a step, they are unable to flex the foot for a normal heel strike, and the toes strike the ground first instead of the heel. This leads to a high stepping gait with the anaesthetic foot being lifted up and dragged with each step, causing painless injuries, ulcers, and florid infections. Tendon transfers to correct the gait do restore the function of the limb, but sadly sensation never returns. The affected anaesthetic limbs remain a potential source of mutilating injuries and infections, and amputation in some cases. Only if meticulous care of the limb is ingrained into patients as second nature will they be trouble free for life. Even then the most careful of patients inevitably develop recurrent injuries that dishearten them.

Tendon transfers are done in leprosy patients whose nerves are paralysed, to restore movement and function to the affected limbs. A functioning tendon is shifted from its original attachment and attached to the tendon of the paralysed muscle to enable the limb to move.

Pain is protective

When the nerve damage causes loss of sensation, the aftermath is grim. If the limb passes through a fireball, it will not wince or pull away as there is no feeling. Even if rodents gnaw at their toes and fingers, patients sleep through it all. Sometimes patients would tell me that when they went to bed, they had all their toes. When they woke up in the morning, some toes were missing after a rodent had done its worst. Many of the patients who waded across rivers to get to the hospital would swear that they had all their toes when they started from one bank. When they reached the other side, blood would be streaming from their injuries. With no sensation on the soles of their feet, they would walk for hours in ill-fitting shoes. Without pain, they develop pressure ulcers on the soles of their feet, which could get infected with maggots.

When we are in pain, do we ever remember to thank God for the protection that pain provides us? *Never!* In all my years as a doctor I have never ever heard a patient, myself included, ever say *Thank God I'm in pain!* We bring the roof down moaning, groaning and popping pills when we are not applying heat and balms to ease the pain. Only leprosy patients wish they could feel pain - to stop, rest and heal.

Fear and Dread

Many of them would tell me about the early skin lesions they ignored, sometimes out of ignorance and sometimes in denial, desperately hoping that it was not leprosy. Many wasted precious time waiting for the tell-tale signs to disappear. Mothers would be frightened to cuddle their babies. *I dare not hold my baby, doctor. How can I feed her? What if she gets it from me?* How sad is that for a new mother waiting to nurse and cuddle her child?

Leprosy destroyed families in unimaginable ways in the early part of the 70s and 80s, bringing in its wake stigma, ostracism and isolation. Until the law was removed in 2019, Leprosy was grounds for divorce in India. A legal ruling changed the law. Could it even hope to change the heart? No one moves away from a patient who apparently looks well but might be nursing an infectious or incurable disease with no tell-tale signs ....but catch anyone willing to sit next to a leprosy patient with facial deformities, a claw hand, a foot drop, or an infected trophic ulcer.

Any chronic illness *especially those with overt tell-tale signs* can trigger a spectrum of mental illnesses, an essential branch of holistic treatment that we did not know well enough to practise except by being supportive, empathetic and amateurish mental hand-holding . Something that troubled Sam and me when we worked with leprosy earlier and Sam when he worked with HIV/AIDS later. We may have helped our patients physically, but we were not even close when treating scars they carried for life. Especially the women who stoically practised the dictum *Ours not to question why, ours but to do and die!*

The Chedithi and the ceramic commode

After internship, Sam and I moved to Karigiri, delighted that Rekha was on the way. My Uncle Eapen and my Aunt Baby, my Mum's younger sister, sibling no. 15, very kindly sent me a live-in maid from Kerala, a middle-aged *Chedithi*, in a traditional *chatta* and *mundu*, to help me during my pregnancy and delivery. We had a tiny one-bedroom suite in the Karigiri guesthouse with a single ensuite bathroom that we shared with the *Chedithi*. There was just one problem. *The Chedithi* had never ever met the western ceramic commode in her life. Whenever she went to the toilet, I would ask her if she had used the flush, and she would reply that she had. I would go in after her and throw up all over the place. In her vocabulary, using the commode meant *to climb up on top of and function*. And flushing merely meant *to put the lid down after use*. My morning sickness spiralled rapidly out of control and threatened to peak into hyperemesis. Meanwhile, when *Chedithi* found out that she was living in the campus of a leprosy hospital, she beat a hasty retreat to Kerala, horrified that she had actually spent a couple of nights there.

An atlas, please

We were delighted when Dr VP Das and his wife, Aunty Beulah, came to visit us in the labour ward when we were waiting for Rekha to arrive. Dr Das, a perfect gentleman with the looks of the film actor Ashok Kumar and a charismatic personality to match, always managed to bring out the best in us as a father figure we loved and respected.

He had come to discuss the bond we had to serve out with the mission. After they made tender enquiries after my health, Dr Das gently broached the subject of the bond. *After a great deal of thought,* he said, *we have decided to send you both to Bhutan*. We had no idea where Bhutan was, but we would have gone to the North Pole if he had asked us. We adored him and were in absolute awe of him. *We'll go,* we said in unison, without even looking at each other. When they got up to leave, Dr Das turned at the door and said, *Susie, I hope you will not have a precipitate delivery when you find out where Bhutan is.* We had to look at an atlas to find out where it was in the Himalayas. It did not matter that it was far from home and all things familiar. It did not matter that we had never climbed a mountain or lived in snow. We were young and enthusiastic. We would have gone anywhere Dr Das sent us. *Anywhere*!

Bhutan

Our first posting in 1973, was to the Gidakom Leprosy Hospital in Khasadrapchu, a few mountain peaks away from Thimphu, the capital of Bhutan. We faced many new and frightening challenges in Bhutan in stark isolation - and survived. We were young and we thought we were invincible, bouncing back from one disaster to another, brushing them aside as challenges that had to be faced as just another day at the office! We would not have survived if it were not for our unswerving faith in God, who had led us without leaving our side. We knew that He was there with us, and we had nothing to fear with Him in our corner holding our hand. We just lived from day to day. We had God, we had each other, and we had Dr VP Das.

Before going to Bhutan, we travelled to Singapore for Rekha's christening at Christ Church. My Dad was retiring, and it was an emotional time for all of us as my Mum and Dad said goodbye to their extended family, the congregation of Christ Church. Saying goodbye to families that had grown up around them for thirty-one years was not an easy task. They were moving out of the parsonage, their home for all those years, ruthlessly discarding memorabilia to downsize as they moved to their own town house in Thomson Ridge. Soon after he helped settle us into my Mum and Dad's new home, Sam left for Bhutan while Rekha and I stayed back, as the Himalayas would have been bitterly cold for the baby in January. The plan was that we would join him in three months when we hoped it would be a little warmer. A few weeks after he landed, Sam sent me a desperate message asking us to join him as he could not stand the loneliness. As long as he was working and busy, the loneliness did not worry him. But, coming home to a cold and empty house, so silent he could hear his own breathing, was driving him nuts. The only sound outside was the howling of the wind that rattled the glass panes of the windows that were shut tight to keep the cold out. *The house,* he wrote, *is a freezing mausoleum!*

The chettan and his chai

We took the first flight out to Calcutta, delighted to be together again. From Calcutta, we flew to Bagdogra and then took the mission Land Rover to Gidakom. Whenever I asked Sam how much further we had to climb, he kept saying, *It's just here... just here,* and I believed him as we sat huddled in the Land Rover for what seemed like eternity. Finally, we stopped at Takhtichu, at 10,000 feet above sea level, for some tea at a small kiosk where the proverbial *mundu*-clad Malayalee *chettan*, one step away from the moon, bundled up in a monkey cap, muffler, and sweater, welcomed us. With astonishing skill, he poured out piping hot tea without spilling a drop, almost as if he was measuring it out in yards between the two steel glasses he held in either hand. I could not believe my eyes when he served us paper crisp *dosa*s, *sambar*, and *vada*s with the tea. He just beamed from ear to ear when I asked him how on earth he managed to get the dosa batter to ferment at that height and temperature.

Dear God, dear God to tsk tsk tsk

After the welcome break, we again bundled up in the Land Rover and continued the climb. The roads going up were narrow winding challenges that managed to simultaneously let traffic up and down the mountain. It was a wonder that there was no sound of metal scraping metal as the vehicles crossed one another! The traffic coming down hugged the curve of the mountain while our Land Rover going up skirted the side of the cliff and a sheer drop of several feet. If a car went down, rescue operations would be futile, I was told. At some spots, I closed my eyes tight, clutched Rekha, who slept through it all, and whispered, *Dear God... Dear God... Dear God,* through clenched teeth. I had no idea what I was praying for. I could not get past the two words *Dear God... Dear God.* All I knew was that if I called on Him, He would get us safely to wherever it was that we were going.

Convinced that this was the last ride we would ever take on earth, the breath-taking beauty of the drive and the driver's skills were wasted on me. I was sure that we were going to hurtle down an unknown mountain into oblivion. Growing up on an island, the only mountains I had ever seen were Fraser's Hill and the Cameron Highlands, holiday destinations in Malaysia. They had both now shrunk to mere pimples on the horizon compared with the mountains of the Himalayas. When I did open my eyes during the journey, the spectacular beauty of the mountains and the wild flowers and foliage took my breath away.

Rhododendrons, poinsettias, and many wild flowers I had never seen before waved out from the lush green cover of the mountainside. Colourful Buddhist prayer flags wafted in the wind welcoming visitors to the ancient Himalayan kingdom with a Zen-like calm and peace. Sometimes a crystal-clear waterfall would break the monotony, gushing and tumbling down the side of the mountain in rainbow colours as the water spray burst in the air. Far in the distance, the snow-capped mountains stood tall and proud as silent witnesses of God's magnificent creation, watching us climb the road cut into the curve of the mountain.

After about nine hours of telling me that it was only a short distance away, Sam finally told me that we had reached Gidakom Hospital. I could not see a thing as I peered out into the pitch-black darkness of the night. How could I when Gidakom had no electricity? A hydel plant supplied a temperamental flicker of light for about two hours in the evening, after which the whole place went to sleep and hurricane lamps lit the emergencies. We creaked and cranked up the last lap and stopped at the dimly lit guesthouse where a crowd of staff and patients was waiting to welcome us. Apparently they had been tracking the headlights of the Land Rover for an hour as it ascended the last lap of the climb. Crowding around, they inspected us from head to toe, holding their lamps high up above their heads. Shaking their heads, they muttered, *Tsk*, and something in Bhutanese that I did not understand. I had no idea what was happening, and neither did Sam.

The next morning, we found out what the *Tsk* was all about. Sam had set up home before we arrived with a few random family photographs on the mantelpiece, some of which were from our wedding album. Apparently, they had seen the photographs on display and were expecting the doctor's slim wife from the wedding photographs to alight daintily from the car. They were taken aback when they saw a person several kilos heavier than the photograph, stiff from bouncing around on the road for hours, roll out of the car bundled up in layers of warm clothes. I believe what they muttered in Bhutanese was, *Poor thing, his first wife must have died, and the doctor-sahib must have married again... tsk tsk tsk...*

We managed to survive our first night in the cold and draughty guesthouse huddled between scratchy blankets that gave us the giggles because they generated static electricity every time we moved. In the middle of the night, Sam turned to me and asked in an extremely serious voice if I wanted to go back to Singapore with the baby. He said that he would stay on in Gidakom and finish the five-year bond. My answer, through frozen lips, is unprintable.

In the morning, when we woke up, our Nepali helper, Kancha, appeared at the door to make tea and breakfast. We washed in ice-cold water and shot out of the bathroom as fast as we could. Migrating to the kitchen, we huddled around the wood fire he stoked and watched him make tea, parathas, and the fluffiest omelettes I have ever seen. Rekha, wrapped in her woollies and cap, gurgled and cooed happily, oblivious to the changes around her. A few weeks later, the incumbent medical superintendent, Dr John Geater, and his family returned to England. When Sam took charge, we moved into the superintendent's residence, an extremely cosy, comfortable, and spacious bungalow.

The kitchen had an Aga stove look-alike. Basically, it was a metal sheet resting on a hollow compartment of bricks that was divided into three sections. Firewood burned in the middle section, heating the metal plate on top. To the left of the firewood compartment was a tank with boiling water, and to its right was a compartment with adjustable racks that could be used as an oven. With time and practice, I learnt which part of the metal plate on top of the burning firewood was hot, which was hotter, and which was hottest. Rearranging the pots, I learnt to cook and keep food warm even as I learned to bake bread and cakes in an oven with no thermostat.

Our home
The Gidakom Leprosy Hospital was set on a quiet hillside near Khasadrapchu, overlooking a river that flowed with rainbow trout. The valley sucked in the passing wind, changing it into an eerie howl to punctuate the placid sound of flowing water. Sometimes the howling wind was the only sound you heard in the still of the night. The colour palette of the quiet hillside changed with the seasons, when the white of the winter snow

melted into the vibrant colours of spring.

Jit Bahadur, a gifted gardener crippled with arthritis, would for most of the year, be on painkillers and in front of the fire in the colder months. We never knew when he did what he did, planting bulbs and seeds to produce the flowers that sprung up to meet us in spring. Miles and miles of multi-coloured cosmos moved like sheets of velvet. Brilliant poppies popped up at you while the chrysanthemums, poinsettias, rhododendrons, violets, pansies, and the fruit blossoms of the apple, the peach, and the plum blazed with dazzling colours. Our house was at a higher level than the hospital, and we would stand mesmerised for hours drinking in the beauty of the hillside, be it the white of the snow or the colours of spring.

The view from the window was magnificent. We looked out at a range of the snow-capped Himalayan mountain peaks that took our breath away every morning. Every other place that we had lived in before Gidakom seemed distant and surreal. I forgot the breaking of waves on the shores of Singapore. I forgot the heat and dust of Vellore. I forgot every other place I had lived in or visited. It almost seemed as if this was the only place on the face of the earth that existed at that point in time.

Baking bread

In the 1970s, Thimphu had just one bakery. The Swiss Bakery, run by an expat, served homemade bread, cakes, and all sorts of delicious pastries. Eventually, after a few fluke hits and disastrous misses, I learnt to bake our own bread. A bread-crazy husband and two toddlers had me revisiting my long-forgotten domestic science classes at St Margaret's, using the warmth of the dying embers of the fireplace to prove the yeast. We had no timers and no oven thermometers to guide us. Sometimes the Aga worked perfectly, and sometimes it did not. Soon Sam, the kids, and visitors to Gidakom, including my Mum and Dad, woke up to the smell of fresh bread wafting from the kitchen. Cheered on by an appreciative audience making encouraging noises, I became bolder with my experiments and went on to bake pastries and biscuits that resembled the glossy pictures in my recipe books. Ultimately, I even mustered enough courage to try the traditional Christmas cake recipe my Mum had followed for years.

Our supply of meat, primarily chicken, came from the cold storage in Thimphu, run by the Hings, a Chinese family settled in Bhutan. The country was in official mourning with the passing of the third King, His Majesty Jigme Dorji Wangchuk, in 1972, and the slaughtering of animals was banned. Animals that fell off the side of the hill were acceptable, and every now and then, an animal would mysteriously fall down the hill, and meat would be sold at the local shop down the road.

Ema Tashi, the national dish of Bhutan, was an acquired taste. A unique brew of butter, goat cheese and green chillies cooked on a slow fire, it warmed parts of our body we had forgotten we had. Deliciously piquant and loaded with calories, it sat for a moment on the lips and forever on the hips. Butter tea, which met us everywhere when we went visiting, was something I never got used to. Sam, not wishing to appear rude, would end up drinking two cups of butter tea, his and mine.

My patients and I

Sam often crossed heights where no doctor had set foot before. When he was away for days on end and incommunicado, I would be alone for weeks, when the staff and patients formed a protective band around Rekha, Anish, and me. Their devotion to our family was quite touching as they surrounded us with a love I cannot describe.

Language was a problem in Bhutan as I never learnt Dzongkha well enough to converse with them. What we lacked in words, we made up with sign language, eye talk, shy smiles, and facial expressions. They would talk to me, and I would listen. I may not have understood Dzongkha, but I understood their emotions, their pain, and their quiet resignation. If I was unwell and could not go down, they would troop up to check on me with anxious faces pressed against my window pane. I learnt many lessons from my patients, valuable lessons that I carry close to my heart. They taught me to look at life realistically, with a sharper perspective and to appreciate the saying: *I cried when I had no shoes, until I saw a man with no legs.*

Anish and the kerosene nightmare

We raised two babies on cloth nappies washed in ice-cold water that did not dry for days on end. As there was no paediatrician close by, we looked after Rekha and Anish when they fell ill. A frightening thought when I look back on our confidence, when so many things could have gone wrong. There were no vaccinations against measles, chickenpox, or mumps. They had them all and so did I, along with them.

We had a frightening medical emergency when Anish was a toddler. He had wandered into the kitchen and picked up a bottle of liquid lying on the floor. Thinking it was water, he drank the kerosene that was used to start the wood stove. I was down at the hospital when it happened, and the maid, in her panic, put her fingers in his throat and made him vomit as much of it as was possible. Unfortunately, he aspirated some of it and developed pneumonia. We started him on antibiotics and rushed him to Calcutta with an overnight stop in Phuntsholing, on what must have been the most terrifying road trip of our lives. Wrapped in blankets and held close to the warmth of our hearts, he was blue and hardly breathing. We thought we had lost him by the time we got to the Bella Vue nursing home in Calcutta. Mercifully, he recovered, and we all returned home safely.

Uncle Sampath Raj

Our earlier days of travel in Bhutan with the kids were nothing short of an expedition since we could get stuck on the road for hours on end in the middle of nowhere because of landslides, snow, or fallen trees. The passengers in the Land Rover would be squashed against pickaxes, shovels, a kerosene stove, kerosene in a jerry can, basic rations, blankets, and all sorts of bric-a-brac in addition to clothes, cloth diapers, and stuffed animals. That was before we met Uncle Sampath Raj, as he was affectionately known, and the BRTF, the Border Road Task Force.

Dotted along the roads of Bhutan were stations of the BRTF manned by the angels who ministered to travellers stranded on the roads. At one of these roadblocks, we met Mr Sampath Raj, who was in charge of the BRTF. He adopted us and kept in touch with our adventures on the road, pointing us to the nearest BRTF post whenever we encountered a roadblock. The kind staff went out of their way to look after us until the block was cleared, serving us a hot meal with rice, *dhal*, and potato. Uncle Sampath Raj would stop by at Gidakom on his official rounds, and we would have a piping hot meal for him with *sambar* for a taste of home food. He will always be remembered in the annals of our family history as the man who brought Bhaji into our lives.

The vegetarian bird

Bhaji, our Man Friday, was an ex-serviceman with the kindest, crinkliest eyes and smile. As I am not from an armed forces background, I never ever got used to him stiffening to attention and clicking his heels when called. When he wished us goodnight before he left for his room, he would come to attention and salute us. This had me jumping up to salute him back, and Sam in splits. He was a faithful and loyal old friend whom we called Bhaji, *grandfather* in Nepali. We were blessed when he chose to share his life with us both in Bhutan, Nepal, and later with my Mum and Dad in Chennai.

When our kids were growing up, we had to invent all sorts of ways of dressing up leftover rice. Undoubtedly, mixed fried rice was a great favourite that appeared with predictable regularity on the table, in their lunch boxes, and on picnics, when we took them down to the river, with Bhaji carrying Anish straddled across his shoulders and Rekha on his hip. They loved Bhaji and really believed that he was their Nepali grandfather.

There were no supermarkets or departmental stores to run to for stuff when guests arrived unannounced, and ordering online was not an option as it had not even been conceptualised. Bhaji and I did not get in a flap; we just sprang into action and improvised, assembling dishes that we served with panache. With time, Bhaji was in total sync with my crazy adventures in our resource-challenged kitchen and took his cue from the look on my face. One afternoon, a top-ranking Indian engineer from a hydel project in Bhutan dropped in unexpectedly just as we were sitting down to dinner. With years of research and development behind me, I swung into *Operation Stretch*. Wasting no time, I thinned the chicken curry, added two boiled and quartered potatoes, salt, and sprinkled a little more cilantro and invited our guest to the dining table. He sat down, took one look at the bits of bird anatomy floating in the gravy, looked up at me, and said very apologetically, *Madam,*

I am a vegetarian. My jaw fell with a loud thud to the floor. I looked at Sam for help, but he was disintegrating rapidly into a heap of acute embarrassment at the other end of the table and deliberately avoiding my eye. Nonchalantly, I smiled as if I was used to vegetarians gawking in shock at birds floating in gravy on the table. Pretending as if this was only the first of many courses, I whisked the offending bird out of sight into the kitchen and offered him the cold *channa* from lunch dressed up as a tantalising *channa chat* starter while I cooked the second of many courses even as he sat at the table. *Ema Tashi* was a lifesaver as we never ran out of the three ingredients that went into it: butter, cheese and chilli. It did not matter if it was cooked in a loud and temperamental pressure cooker that whistled off-key in the kitchen as guests sat at the dining table in the next room. A hack that Bhaji and I used in dire straits was spring rolls filled with leftover fried rice. This was an all-time favourite when served hot. Bhaji, meanwhile, had swung silently into action, without a spoken word between us, as he started kneading the dough for spring roll wrappers. Deftly, he rolled them out into thin squares and filled them with small quantities of fried rice that were left over from the kids' lunch and fried them crisp on the old Aga stove. We arranged the rolls like a clock face with a small bowl of tomato sauce in the centre, and I sashayed into the dining room with the curtain-raiser.

After an entertaining meal and several helpings of seconds later, the polite official rose from the table, totally amused. He thanked us at the door and said that he had never tasted such crisp and tasty spring rolls in all his field trips in the snow-capped mountains.

The earth moved

Once when Sam was away on one of his field trips, we had a downpour of torrential rain. On the third day the rains stopped. Delighted, I ran to the foyer of the house to open the front door and got the shock of my life. The house was standing apart on land separated from the front lawn by a yawning chasm about three feet wide with a sheer drop of ten to fifteen feet! The three steps leading down to the lawn from the front door were suspended in the air. If I had stepped out, it would have been disastrous as Anish, five months in utero, and I would have fallen all the way down. Mercifully, the front door opened inside and did not swing out when opened. My hand was still on the doorknob, and my feet were still inside the house. The house had been built on one level, and the dip in the land had been filled with earth, which moved when the landslide shook the place.

Closing the front door, I ran to the back door and found to my utter relief that no earth had moved at the back of the house. The steps were in place and led straight onto the grass verge of the backyard. By then, the patients and staff had gathered around the house to survey the damage. They contacted Mr Philippose, an engineer from Kerala who was working with the hydel project down the road. Extremely kind and always helpful, he charged up the hill with men, machines, and mud to fill the defect in front of the house. When they finished a few hours later, there was no trace of the chasm, and the three steps once again connected to the front lawn.

That night I developed premature contractions. I sat up in bed wondering if I should call Dr Norbu, the obstetrician at Thimphu General Hospital. It was around midnight, and I thought I would give her a call in the morning and lay down again, trying to sleep. Around 3 am, the contractions started increasing in duration and intensity. Alarmed, I got out of bed and hobbled to the medicine box that I kept in the house for emergencies. In my anxiety, I must have fumbled. Before I knew it, the contents of the box were on the floor. Gingerly, I lowered myself down, clutching my abdomen, which had suddenly upped its beat and started doing its own thing. I found the ampoule of Pethidine and injected it into my right thigh, just as I had seen diabetic patients do with insulin. Too frightened to move, I sat on the floor with my back against the wall stroking my abdomen for what seemed like a lifetime. To keep my sanity, I kept coaxing Anish-in-utero to stay inside like a good boy as it was not time yet. The thought of a premature baby in Gidakom conjured up all sorts of horrific visuals that left me chanting my favourite mantra, *dear God, dear God, dear God.* Mercifully, Rekha, who was lying in her crib, slept through it all, and the contractions eventually became less intense. At 6 am, I rang Dr Norbu and told her the events of the night. She was extremely kind and promised to come and see me as soon as she could. She had a terrible time coming to Gidakom as bits of the road had caved in, and vehicles were plying dangerously on planks that bridged the yawning gaps. A sight for sore eyes, she braved it all and arrived in her jeep. She examined me and reassured me that all was well, put me on some medication, and left to rush back to her OPD. I will never ever forget her kindness. I settled down as she had predicted and went back to work after a few days. I carried Anish to term and went back to CMC for his birth.

There was no way of letting Sam know about the adventures at Gidakom. When he returned a few days later, someone met him in Thimphu and said, *So sorry to hear about your house, doctor.* His heart sank because he had no clue what had happened. When they continued with, *so sorry to hear about your wife, doctor,* his heart sank further. When he finally reached home, he told me that he had no idea how he drove from Thimphu to Gidakom, not knowing what awaited him on arrival.

My first bear maul
My first bear maul in Bhutan was on a night in 1973 which I will never forget. The declared period of mourning for the late King prohibited hunting and fishing in the kingdom. A hunting party had gone up the hill on the opposite bank defying the ban. The gall bladders and bile of bears contain high levels of ursodeoxycholic acid, which is harvested and used in traditional medicine to treat a host of diseases. It is also used in toothpaste, facial cleansers, masks for acne, wine, and gourmet tea. Some even use it as an aphrodisiac when all else fails.

The poachers spotted a bear in the woods. Unfortunately, they did not kill it outright despite the volley of bullets fired. The bear, who sustained multiple injuries, prowled around wounded, sore, and angry. In pain, it fell upon and attacked an unsuspecting villager in the early hours of the morning when he had stepped outside to relieve himself. The poachers following the wounded bear took pot shots as man and bear rolled down the hill. Some bullets went into the bear, and some into the man. Finally, all was still and the bear lay dead on top of the human, who had passed out in fear, totally squashed under its weight. When they prised the dead bear away from the man, they realised that the man needed immediate medical aid as he was badly injured and barely alive.

This posed a major problem as they could not take the injured man to any of the government hospitals in Thimphu for treatment. They would have had some serious explaining to do within prison walls. So, they brought him down to the leprosy hospital on a lonely hill in Khasadrapchu.

Sam was away on tour, and I was seven months pregnant with our son, Anish. The adventures that I shared with Anish-in-utero (*and out!*) would fill another book! The staff used to joke that it seemed as if all the complex cases came only on the nights that the *doctor-sahib* was away on tour. When he was at home, we never seemed to have disturbed nights or complicated cases and got to sleep peacefully through the night. The minute his vehicle disappeared down the hill, all sorts of nocturnal emergencies would arrive as if on cue. When they woke me up, I struggled to focus on what they were saying. *Doctor Memsahib, come soon, come soon… They've brought a bear maul for treatment. His face is in bad shape; come soon.* I had never treated a bear maul in my life. No, correct that to I had never seen a bear in my life and only read about bear mauls in my youth. Slightly apprehensive, I got dressed and rushed down to the hospital, not knowing what I would find. The first person I met was the irate wife of the injured man. Incensed with grief, anger and fear, she was attacking her husband, shrieking hysterically. *Aiyee… Aiyee…,* she wailed as she flailed him with both her hands. The patient was cowering in a corner, a scarf covering his face and a large, checked blanket covering his thin frame as he shivered and shook. He kept begging the staff to keep her away from him. The bear maul was nothing compared to his wife's wrath. *Save me, save me,* he moaned. His speech was slurred and he reeked of the local hooch, a popular painkiller in the hills. We managed to get her out of the room, lock the door and lay him on the table. Meanwhile, the nurses and theatre staff sprang into action and got their act together like a well-tuned orchestra. They found a vein on his limp forearm to start the IV drip, added the antibiotic after a test dose, gave him an anti-tetanus shot, and got the primitive suction machine whirring. I did not know what to expect and was appalled to see his face when they removed the dirty, blood-stained scarf that covered it. I have never seen anything so macabre in my entire life. His face was a bloody mess. Jagged strips of skin hung in shreds around his face, trickling blood onto the green sterile sheet. Mercifully, his nose, eyes, and ears were spared. There were no injuries near his bloodshot eyes that looked imploringly up at me. The facial wounds were superficial but teeming with short black bear hairs swimming in blood. I did not know where to start. We spent a long time cleaning the wounds, irrigating them meticulously with saline. The patient had passed out, too inebriated to care or feel any pain. I managed to put eighty-one sutures in his face for what must have been several hours, perched on a revolving metal stool with Anish-in-utero between the injured man and me.

He had a couple of bullets embedded in his back and arms, which we managed to remove. Unfortunately, one of the bullets embedded in the popliteal fossa of the right knee was quite deep and inaccessible. After repairing his face, we immobilised the limb in a Thomas splint and shifted him and his wife in the hospital Land Rover to the Indian Military Training Team (IMTRAT) Hospital at Haa for advanced orthopaedic care. It was a long and bumpy ride to Haa, but there was no way we could send him to any hospital in Thimphu, which undoubtedly would have been nearer.

The face endowed with a good blood supply healed well, and he came back a few weeks later with his grateful wife and a lopsided smile. Only a few stitches in the buccal mucosa had gaped and needed re-suturing on a follow-up visit. Repaired and reconstructed, he was a far cry from the terrified human being I had met on that fateful night. We had many wild animal mauls after that. Bears go for the face while the big cats like the cheetah and the leopard go for the throat. However,

I have never met anything as blood curdling as my first bear maul in Bhutan.

Sam the traveller

Sam has always been the traveller in our lives. He did the village outreach programme while I worked at the hospital. He would set off with the paramedics and supplies to seek out the leprosy patients who had defaulted and never showed up for follow-ups or medication. This was no easy task as some patients gave false names and addresses, making the entire exercise a frustrating waste of time. It did, however, give Sam a chance to understand what the paramedics were up against in terms of travail, travel, and terrain. Some villages were mountains apart and took several days to reach. Sometimes they had to cross rivers in the rains when the paramedics carried him on their back. Clothes and socks washed in salt prevented leeches from hanging onto them, but every time they crossed a river, a bit of the salt would wash off. Eventually, there would be no salt left to ward off the leeches.

When he came back home, Sam would shed most of his clothes and footwear in a tub outside filled with salt water to kill off the leeches before he went in for a shower. Sometimes this would be the first bath he had in a long while.

He would come back with stories of people and lifestyles untouched by time. When he trekked to Bhumthang, he met a group of people with a polyandrous matriarchal system where women managed to very successfully juggle several husbands at the same time. People in Bhumthang did not use money but bartered fruit and vegetables for paper, salt and provisions. Modern gadgets and gizmos had not made inroads into Bhutan. Legend has it that when the first automobile drove up the road, villagers thought it was a beast of burden and offered it fodder.

The Bhutanese were a happy and peaceful lot who lived simple and uncomplicated lives with low levels of stress.

Gidakom Hospital

As Gidakom Hospital was the only hospital for many hills around, we started a general clinic to treat people of the nearby villages. Word soon spread, and people from the surrounding villages made tentative tracks to the hospital seeking medical aid, including obstetric care, albeit extremely cautiously, conscious of the stigma associated with leprosy. With time, the stigma associated with the disease and the hospital diminished, and the villagers knew that they would be helped if they came to us. What we could not handle, we referred to Dr Norbu and Dr (Mrs) Norbu, who ran the Thimphu General Hospital with a team of specialists and a full-fledged operation theatre.

The leprosy patients at Gidakom Hospital were admitted to the male and female medical and surgical wards at the foot of the hill. The medical wards had patients with type 1 and type 2 Lepra reactions. The surgical wards had patients who needed long-term ulcer care. If I close my eyes, I can hear our patients crying in pain. Something I heard a lot less in later years when treatment modalities for neuritis improved. As leprosy patients were not readily accepted in general hospitals, they gravitated to Gidakom when they fell ill, confident that they would be looked after. No patient who reached Gidakom Hospital was ever turned away.

For many of them, this was the only home that they had known in a very long time. In the wards, they had a warm bed with blankets, running water and three meals a day. They were not outcasts. They were with other human beings with similar problems. When they became better, they were understandably reluctant to leave the comfort zone of the hospital, and they resisted discharge. Many had left their own homes, never to return again. Some returned to their homes, peering in as outsiders, or stayed in pigsties outside their homes, grateful for the crumbs that came their way as they accepted rejection as a way of life. Very few had loving and understanding families to return to. Some patients, when they were discharged, moved into makeshift huts that sprung up as satellite settlements at the periphery of the hospital. Patients formed easy liaisons of convenience and started families of their own. I was amazed at their cheerful acceptance of rejection, their fortitude in pain, and their calm in the face of disaster. They learnt to live life on their own terms, sad terms, hard terms perhaps, but their own terms.

The Gidakom Hospital staff were a quiet and dignified bunch of caregivers who looked after the patients with a dedication that humbled us. Many had made Gidakom their home. The nursing superintendent, Mr M Sangma, was from Assam. Rongong, the physiotherapist, and his wife, Deepti, had served the hospital all their lives. Deepti's sister Kunti, also a nurse, was married to Peter, who ran the pharmacy. Tshering Doma, a lovely Bhutanese nurse, was a ray of sunshine in the ward. Cheerful and smiling, I have never ever heard her say no to any extra work. Ever. She was someone who walked the extra mile for the patients, and we all loved her. Kaka, a Bhutanese paramedic, led a dedicated team of paramedics who scoured the mountains searching for new leprosy patients and for old patients who had defaulted on treatment. The dedication of the staff was the glue that kept the hospital together as they welcomed leprosy patients from all over Bhutan.

Meals for the patients were cooked in the main kitchen and sent out to be served in the wards in big vessels. Rice was the staple diet, with lentils and vegetables. The locally grown potato and radish were readily available and great favourites. A dish they enjoyed immensely was *Ema Tashi*. Chicken, mutton, or pork, served twice a week, was a treat they looked forward to. The cooks were a cheerful lot and knew precisely what appealed to the patients' palate. The gravy had to be fiery, spicy, and chilli hot. Every day, the faithful kitchen staff churned out meals like clockwork for the patients, whether it rained or snowed. At lunchtime, the head cook would find me, wherever I was in the hospital, with the flavour of the day in a wooden ladle. This was a routine we established. I would stop whatever I was doing, push up my glasses, and inspect the gravy before I smelt it and tasted it. Sometimes I would pretend to frown and make faces at the contents of the spoon and look up at him disapprovingly. Sometimes I gave him a thumbs up and rolled my eyes in delight. Thanks to this game of charades, they were a little careful about cooking for the patients and kept up with the song-and-dance routine of inspection that we had going. Sometimes the patients would go fishing for rainbow trout in the river below and give it to the cooks in the kitchen to make a curry. Like all good anglers, they returned with stories of the ones that got away, and with every telling, their arms would move out a fraction of an inch wider.

Obstetrics in a leprosy hospital

I remember quite vividly the first obstetric case and delivery we conducted in the hospital. Neither of the baby's parents were leprosy patients. The baby's father was a teacher at the Tibetan school, and his wife, a young Tibetan girl, barely out of her teens, was too far gone in labour to be shifted anywhere when they brought her to the hospital late in the evening. We had no choice but to deliver the baby, our first normal delivery in the Gidakom Leprosy Hospital.

Deepti, Kunti, and Tshering Doma prepped the patient

and Mr M Sangma and Rongong prepped the treatment room next to the office in the main building. It was freezing cold, and we felt desperately sorry for the patient, who had to bare it all without an electric heater. To heat the room, we fired up a *bukhari*, the traditional space heater, which in reality is a wood-burning metal stove placed in the centre of the room. The heat generated from the firewood heats a room, while a metal chimney removes the smoke.

More than the lack of facilities surrounding the birth of a child in Gidakom Hospital, the *bukhari* burning firewood next to the patient's bed terrified me. It reminded me of the many deaths I had certified in the camps housing migrant labour working on the hydel project near the hospital. The labourers would be found lying dead on the floor in the morning. They would go to bed with the *bukhari* burning in a room with all the windows closed to keep the cold out. In the night, the fire would go out and the smouldering embers would give off the poisonous carbon monoxide, a heavy gas that sinks low in a room killing animals and people sleeping on the floor. All sorts of disastrous possibilities flashed in my mind, grim enough to keep me awake throughout the night, watching the *bukhari* in the centre of the makeshift labour room.

Actually, none of us slept that night as Deepti, Kunti, Tshering Doma, and I kept vigil. When we were not checking the patient's vitals, abdomen, and sanitary pad, we were checking to see if the *bukhari* was still active. Not for a second did we take our eyes off the baby we had wrapped in several blankets. We took turns holding the baby through the whole night, sitting as far away from the *bukhari* as possible, amazed as always by the miracle of childbirth and the entry of a new baby into the world, while the exhausted mother slept blissfully, glad for the rest. This became a pattern as the stigma of leprosy diminished with time, and obstetric cases were admitted freely to the leprosy hospital. The staff and the leprosy patients, ringside and totally involved, cheered as they rejoiced with the parents at the first cry of a normal baby born in their hospital.

We managed obstetric care under suboptimal conditions without any pregnancy loss and maternal death – *only* because we were never alone . The Omnipresent was always there with us at every birth.

The delivery cases were admitted to a stark room with a metal obstetric bed and two wooden cots, one for the patient in labour and one for me. Unfortunately, there was no running hot water to clean up after the delivery and I used to feel desperately sorry for the mother who lay there on the cold metal bed with a thin plastic mattress, completely exhausted after her ordeal. However, the moment the baby was placed in her arms, the tiredness would disappear like magic when she nestled the baby close to her breast and mother and child bonded. The light in a mother's eyes when she meets her infant for the first time, can light up the darkest nights of the North Pole and then some. The rest of us in the room always felt like voyeurs intruding on their epiphany mother-child moment.

We never threw the placenta away. The placenta is a highly specialised nutrient-rich tissue that is immunologically privileged. The amniotic membrane is known to act as an allograft with healing properties in wound care. We used them as adjuvant therapy in wound care to promote soft tissue healing for the recalcitrant non-healing ulcers of leprosy patients, with appreciable results.

Bhutan's first eye camp

In the early 1970s, Bhutan had an elderly population who were sight-challenged because of cataracts in various stages of maturity. Responding to the need, Sam wrote to Dr Anna Thomas, our professor at the Schell Eye Hospital of the Christian Medical College and Hospital, Vellore. When we did not hear from her we assumed that she was not coming. One morning, out of the blue, the postman brought a letter from Dr Anna Thomas informing us that she and her team were arriving in two weeks. We were absolutely delighted!

As students, we had attended the eye camps she conducted in villages with her team, restoring sight to the villagers with minimal fuss and bother. The team would start work in the evening, using the darkness of the night to do the screening that would normally have been done in a dark room in a hospital. Patients would be prepped for surgery in the morning when Sister Soshamma, who had worked with Dr Thomas for decades and knew her every move, would place the correct instrument in her outstretched hand. As did Somu, the paramedic who accompanied them everywhere. The legendary threesome orchestrated a magnum opus to restore sight to the sightless. If Sister Soshamma was Dr Anna Thomas' right hand, Somu was her left as they set up multiple operating beds. Dr Anna Thomas would move from table to table, scrubbed and gloved, to operate while Sister Soshamma and Somu bandaged and dressed the cases she operated on. With years of R&D they had perfected a flawless modus operandi to minimize untoward incidents and infections. The carefully screened cases were operated on under stringent sterile conditions.

Sam ran around and got all the official paperwork done in record time and set to work revamping the empty Khasadrapchu School building at the end of the Gidakom Road. After several coats of fresh paint, the building was sanitised and declared ready. Why they even had a couple of new toilets put in!

Lyonpo Dawa Tshering, the Foreign Minister of Bhutan,

inaugurated the first eye camp and dedicated it to the memory of the late third King of the Druk Kingdom, His Majesty Druk Gyalpo Jigme Dorji Wangchuck, the benevolent monarch the nation remembered with great love and affection. The government extensively publicised the event and many trekked for miles from remote villages to Gidakom in search of sight. Some patients were carried on the back of a younger relative while others were brought in baskets. The eye camp ran for a week and all those with operable cataracts returned home sighted and aware, to a new life with glasses provided free of cost by the Govt of Bhutan. Word soon spread that Gidakom Leprosy Hospital looked after general patients too – it was not just another leprosy hospital, and it was not such a bad place after all.

Poisonous berries on payday

On the night Dr Anna Thomas and her team arrived, there was an unprecedented upheaval, the likes of which had never been seen before in Gidakom Hospital. Twelve labourers, all male of different ages, were brought in with poisoning. On payday, the homesick migrant labour contracted for construction work from far and distant places would swig *Chaang*, a Tibetan beverage. *Chaang*, low in its alcohol content, tasted like ale and produced an intensely happy feeling of warmth and well-being dispelling their loneliness in the cold night. If they inadvertently plucked and ate the wild berries that grew on the wayside as they wandered home, the berries would react with the *Chaang* to release a neurotoxin that caused opisthotonos. This is an abnormal posture due to the spasms of the extensor muscles of the neck, trunk, and lower extremities with severe backward arching from neck to heel. With the trunk elevated a few inches, only the back of the head and the heel would touch the bed when they lay flat - extremely scary for the patient and the onlooker!

Leaving Dr Thomas to rest, Sam and I ran down to the OPD, with Sister Soshamma and Somu following close on our heels. There was utter confusion in the OPD, with the labour and their supervisors yelling and shouting. This was the first time that we had so many cases of poisoning in a single night. Men of all shapes and sizes lay arched with only the back of their heads and their toes touching the ground. Somu and Sister Soshamma were brilliant. Rolling up their sleeves, they pitched in, and in no time, multiple units of gastric lavage were set up.

Lanky and loose-limbed, Somu, a look-alike of Nagesh, the comedian of yesteryears on the Tamil screen, was a natural comic. He spoke no Hindi and the labourers spoke no Tamil. We were in splits seeing him sit purposefully astride cowering labourers urging them in colloquial Tamil to relax while he passed tubes down their throats. *Dai, vaai thora da, Dai, Dai, Dai... Pallu kaattathe Da... Dai Pallukadikathe Da... Dai, Dai...*, which translates to *Boy, Boy, open your mouth... don't show me your teeth, Boy, Boy don't bite your teeth, Boy, Boy!* Soon, the inebriated men were retching and gagging all over the place, emptying the poisonous contents of their stomachs and lying flat, exhausted and limping towards recovery. Trudging down the hill later that night, the exhilarated duo, Sister Soshamma and Somu, both agreed that they had not had such excitement in a long, long time. Sam and I, had also never had such an exciting and entertaining night in a long while!

The coronation of the 4th King of Bhutan

When His Majesty Jigme Dorji Wangchuk, the third King of Bhutan, passed away on 21st July 1972 in Nairobi at the age of forty-five, his only son, the Crown Prince, HRH Jigme Singye Wangchuk, ascended the throne to become the fourth King of Bhutan. The coronation took place when he was eighteen years old, making him the youngest ruling monarch in the world. Sam and I were honoured royal guests, as were my Mum and Dad who were visiting us at that time. The spectacular event held in Thimphu and attended by dignitaries from all over the world, lasted three days. Buddhist priests and lamas successfully prayed away the rain clouds that threatened to dampen the coronation and the ceremony took place, as scheduled, under sunny skies, on the crisp morning of 2nd June 1974, with the yellow-and-orange flag of Bhutan flying high. With a ringside view of the epic once-in-a-lifetime event, we watched a young man wise beyond his years claim his birthright as the monks placed the Raven Crown of Bhutan on his head.

HM Jigme Singye Wangchuk cared deeply for the leprosy patients in Gidakom Hospital. He kept abreast of the growth and progress of the hospital through regular visits his mother, HM Ashi Kesang Choden Wangchuck and his sister HRH Ashi Dechen Wangmo Wangchuk, made to Gidakom Hospital. The Royal Family with its encouragement and unstinting support of all the new projects, contributed immensely to the improvement of the hospital and the well-being of the patients.

With time, the Fourth King of Bhutan assumed the responsibility of leading the landlocked kingdom forward with a careful balance of tradition and modernization, making it one of the youngest democracies in the world. Assisted ably by his ministers and the Gross National Happiness Commission, the young visionary monarch worked tirelessly to change the lives of the people of Bhutan by introducing the term Gross National Happiness, GNH, a philosophy that includes an index to measure the collective happiness of the country's population to guide the policies of the government. These work to increase the happiness and well-being of people while zealously protecting their traditions and environment.

The coronation gold medal

During the coronation celebrations, Sam was awarded a gold medal in appreciation of his meritorious services in the care and treatment of leprosy patients in the kingdom of Bhutan. We acknowledged it as recognition for the entire team at the hospital: all the dedicated nurses, physiotherapists, and ward staff who looked after the patients in the hospital. Not forgetting all the dedicated paramedics who risked their lives in search of patients who were too ill, frightened, or disabled to travel to the hospital to get their medicines on time. The staff of Gidakom Leprosy Hospital, the unsung heroes of the 1970s, were an exceptional band of committed caregivers. A team that toiled so tirelessly for the health and well-being of leprosy patients from all over Bhutan.

HM the Queen Mother
Ashi Kesang Choden Wangchuk

On their visits to the Hospital, Her Majesty the Queen Mother, Ashi Kesang Choden Wangchuk, and the King's sister, HRH Ashi Dechen Wangmo Wangchuk, who was in charge of the Ministry for Development would stop by each bed to listen to the stories of the patients, clearly moved by the atrocities that they had suffered in their homes. The empathy of the royal visitors was a great source of comfort to the patients, especially the women. The secretaries who accompanied the royal visitors were commissioned to investigate and report back with sustainable solutions wherever possible. The Queen Mother is one of the most compassionate people I have ever met in my life. Beautiful, cultured, and extremely intelligent, she was interested in the latest treatment modalities available for leprosy patients and would ask to be briefed about the current advances in their treatment whenever she met Sam. Extremely artistic, she sent artisans from Thimphu to paint the internal walls of the newly constructed Community Hall with earth colours, similar to the paintings on the cloth wall hangings, the *Thangka*s. The murals that covered entire walls depicted popular Bhutanese folklore that the patients were familiar with and had them entertained for hours. When the new school building was completed, the paintings that decorated the walls were appropriately child-friendly and colourful.

Patient compliance was a huge problem in the mountains, with many of them failing to regularly take Dapsone. Acedapsone, a long-acting injectable derivative of Dapsone that assured effective blood levels for a hundred days, had been used successfully in other mountainous places such as Papua New Guinea. Sam was convinced that the long-acting drug would be invaluable in the treatment and care of leprosy patients in Bhutan's remote and poorly accessible parts. When Sam updated HM the Queen Mother about the advantages of the injectable form of Dapsone in a mountain terrain like Bhutan, the Queen Mother left no stone unturned in getting Acedapsone for the people of Bhutan. Cost never entered the equation as patients always came first. Completely supportive of the hospital's outreach programme, the Queen Mother sent her personal staff and experienced trekkers to help Sam and the paramedics cut to the chase.

Apples are cash crops that grow well in Bhutan. The Queen Mother donated two thousand apple saplings—a mix of the red, golden, and royal delicious varieties from her personal orchards—to be planted on the higher slopes of the hospital campus for the patients and as an added source of income for the hospital. I remember well the morning we planted the apple orchards in Gidakom. A minister from the government of Bhutan was deputed to initiate the planting. Dressed in a Gho, the national dress for men, he planted the first sapling as his staff sang a song acapella. He danced around the planted sapling with heavy thumping steps in his sports shoes to secure the ground around the sapling. He then invited the patients and staff to do likewise. That morning everyone had a wonderful time planting the saplings and stomping around them, supervised by Her Majesty's orchard staff.

The Queen Mother knowing that I stayed alone with Rekha and Anish when Sam was on his field trips, would send me piles of glossy magazines from the Palace together with all sorts of candy treats for the kids and me. A thoughtful gesture from a kind-hearted lady who cared, a gracious queen who touched the lives of all the people she came in contact with, mine included. The magazines were a welcome distraction; I read and reread them over and over again because there was no other entertainment those days. No phone, no newspaper, no radio and no television. Nor were there friends or family to hang out with when Sam was away. Letters took forever to arrive, and phone calls were never an option. I will never ever forget the Queen Mother or her kindness to me.

Dr Victor Preetam Das
One person we remember with gratitude, respect and the fondest of memories is Dr VP Das, the Leprosy Mission -TLM- Secretary for SE Asia. He was a pillar of support and a mentor who nurtured us. A true leader who led by example, he taught us a great deal more than Leprosy. He taught us how to face life wherever we are planted – even as novices shouldering

tremendous responsibilities in a far and distant land. His unwavering faith in us never failed to give us the courage to meet the challenges. We waited for his letters from TLM's head office in Delhi which used to take almost a month to arrive. One letter from him was all we needed to keep us going till the next one came like clockwork, on time every time. He never treated us like a boss. He remained a compassionate father figure who trusted us, encouraged us and always brought out the best in us. On his regular visits to Bhutan, he lived with us in our modest home on a snowy mountain top, in undeniably humble circumstances. He shared our joys, our sorrows and the challenges we faced. Why he even ate the burnt offerings that I served him as if he enjoyed it!

Dear, dear Dr Das, we will never forget you.

Nepal

We went on to do our postgraduate studies after we finished our term in Bhutan. When Sam completed his DTM&H (Diploma in Tropical Medicine and Hygiene), MSc (Clinical Tropical Medicine), and PhD in London in 1979, we were posted to the Anandaban Leprosy Hospital in Kathmandu. Sam's brief was to start a leprosy research centre in Nepal; however, we had no clue what awaited us when we landed in Kathmandu.

The Nepal we knew in the late '70s was a land of many surprises. The rustic footpaths that led into the interiors and far from the madding crowd, boasted quietly of a land untouched by time and tide, where the tolerant native Nepalese stood out as a race known for their inherent honesty, loyalty and integrity. The Nepal that grew up around the bigger cities, especially Kathmandu, in sharp contrast, was a melting pot of cultures from India, China, Bhutan, the Far East, and the West. The flower children of the 1960s had come and gone, leaving behind a trail of free love and dope. The Tibetans, with their quiet dignity, held on tenaciously to their culture, traditions, and dreams of returning home to Tibet one day. The Indians brought Bollywood and Hindi pop songs, commerce, and trade. Kathmandu attracted the Indian tourist in search of imported goods across the linear porous Indo-Nepal border. To the *nouveau riche*, the casino at the Soaltee Oberoi was Shangri-La and Las Vegas rolled into one - a place to gamble away the rupee. Western tourists in Bermuda shorts, flip flops, carrying cloth tote bags wandered about the markets in search of local vegetables and fruits. On hearing the price of the farm produce, they would do a quick mental conversion to their currency and then turn in surprise to their companions and say *damn cheap*, which earned them the nickname *Damn Cheap Sahibs*. The younger populace preferring faded denim jeans and T-shirts to the traditional Nepali national dress and cap, listened to western pop songs blaring from pirated CDs.

Hinduism was a fragile religious thread that linked India and Nepal. The Pashupatinath temple drew Indian pilgrims throughout the year as did the Indian temples that the Nepalese visited when there was a death in the family. After the cremation ceremony, supervised by the head priests who were Adigas from India, the ashes of their loved ones would be taken to India to be immersed in the holy waters. A prepubescent, blemish-free young girl was chosen from the Newar community after a rigorous selection process to be worshipped and glorified as the Goddess Taleju, the tutelary deity of the Malla Dynasty and the Shah Dynasty. The Living Goddess, as she was known, lived in the Kumari Ghar overlooking the Durbar Square. The Kings of Nepal would visit her for her blessings but they would never visit the open-air Budhanilkantha Temple with its five-metre-long, black basalt statue of the reclining Lord Vishnu in a recessed pool of water. Simply because the reigning King of Nepal was worshipped as a reincarnation of the deity.

Anandaban, the forest of joy

Anandaban Hospital, situated in a pine-scented forest on top of the Himalayas, is undoubtedly one of the most beautiful places on the planet. It is also the last stop for leprosy patients with varying degrees of disabilities, deformities, and comorbidities. Treated as outcasts in their homes, leprosy patients were sometimes deposited with stain and stigma at the Anandaban Leprosy Hospital and forgotten forever. Others swam rivers against the tide and crawled uneven miles on anaesthetic limbs, looking for shelter, medicine, food, acceptance, and the hope of survival; they knew they would receive all this if they made it to the Anandaban Leprosy Hospital.

Artificial limb

We were blessed when Sharan Prasad Ruchal joined the staff. A highly skilled paramedic from Tansen in western Nepal, he doubled up as an anaesthetic technician when needed. Trained in prosthetics at the famous Foot and the Prosthetic Limb Centre in Jaipur, he set up a memorable milestone in patient care when we opened the artificial limb centre in the Anandaban Leprosy Hospital. A man of few words, Ruchal was an invaluable assistant I could depend on with my eyes closed. I admired his integrity, quiet dignity, proficiency at work, and the way he switched effortlessly from one role to another, be it in theatre, in the wards, crafting a limb, or leading the community worship at prayers as their beloved Ruchal Dai.

When we fitted Ram Bahadur with the Jaipur foot after his below-knee amputation, it was to help him move from point A to point B and to give him the confidence and independence he needed as an amputee. It did get Ram Bahadur from point A to point B, but it got him much more than mobility. When he returned after a long gap, we did not recognise him. This was not the patient who had shuffled away gratefully. He now walked with an exaggerated swagger with multiple gold chains and rings glinting from his flamboyant avatar.

After a few swigs from his hip flask, he bragged about how he had made it big to an extremely curious audience, me included. Nepal and India share a long and porous border with multiple check posts that do very little to curb the illegal traffic of humans and drugs in and out of either country. A shrewd entrepreneur, Ram Bahadur devised a novel use for his hollow Jaipur foot. He used to layer the bottom of the hollow limb with hashish wrapped in plastic bags. Over the hashish he would pack raw meat that he allowed to decay. When the stench became unbearable, he would strap the artificial limb back on and hobble across to the check post. Smelling him before they saw him, the guards would pinch their noses and wave him through, presuming that the stench came from his disease. Safely across the border and out of sight, he would empty the contents of his artificial limb, clean it out, and proceed to peddle his wares. Artificial limbs suddenly took on a new meaning with Ram Bahadur's entrepreneurial skills - *you walk with some and you mint with some!*

Shanta Maya

Shanta Maya's husband threw her into the pigsty near the gate of their home when she was diagnosed with leprosy. Without a backward glance or an ounce of remorse, he trotted off and got himself a second wife years younger than him. Shanta Maya never complained. Grateful that she was near her children, she continued to pick up all the crumbs thrown in her direction. With time, her anaesthetic hands clawed, her foot dropped, and she developed ulcers that became infected. She was never taken to any hospital for treatment as she was *persona non grata* - a nuisance and a liability.

Finally, when the overpowering stench from the infected limb was too much to bear, she was thrown out of the pigsty and left on the road. Her youngest son, Kancha, a mere boy of ten who would not be separated from his helpless mother, carried her all the way to Anandaban on his back. Examination revealed that her infected leg could not be salvaged and that she needed a below-knee amputation. Convinced that we did not have the wherewithal to look after her, we decided to send her to the UMN's (United Mission to Nepal) Shanta Bhavan Hospital in Patan, which was undoubtedly better equipped to handle her surgery and post-op care. However, Shanta Maya had other ideas. She had no intention of leaving Anandaban. When the ambulance drew up, we put her in the back seat through one door. No sooner was that done when she would roll out of the other door, grinning mischievously, helped by a willing accomplice, her son Kancha. This happened a few times till we gave in and carried her back to the ward. Shanta Maya had her way, and we did the amputation in Anandaban. Mercifully, the infection was controlled and she survived. A few months later, Sharan Prasad Ruchal, fitted her with a prosthetic limb. The resigned look that she had at admission was gone and she looked immensely happier as she walked around confident about a second chance at life. We loved her from the day she arrived with her quiet dignity. Self-conscious about the gaps in her dental line, Shanta Maya always covered her mouth with her clawed hand whenever she spoke or smiled. We never had lengthy conversations, but I knew she was there smiling sweetly at me; and I knew that she would go back to the ward only after I left the hospital.

Not once did she complain about her lot in life. Nor did she complain about her obnoxious husband or rile against God. She never resorted to imprecatory psalms or pity parties. She just faced life with patience, fortitude, and her unforgettable brand of dignity. Some patients leave us with indelible images and lessons etched in our soul. Some teach us lessons that keep us humbled and grounded. Shanta Maya did just that. Courage has many faces. Shanta Maya's is one of them.

Ramesh, the trapeze artiste
I met Ramesh, the trapeze artiste from Kerala when the circus came to Kathmandu. Walking into the clinic, he gave me a shy smile and asked if I spoke Malayalam. When I replied in Malayalam, he was delighted. We chatted for a while. When the small talk of hearth and home in Kerala, *Veedu evideya, Naadu evideya*, was out of the way, he told me that he was a trapeze artiste in a circus. Then his voice broke and I was stunned when I heard him whisper, *I think I have leprosy*.

Married to a fellow trapeze artist, they had perfected a brilliant act in the circus ring that put food on the table for their toddlers. Recently, he had noticed a hypo pigmented patch on his right arm – an area lighter than his skin colour. The tips of his fingers were becoming progressively numb, and he was petrified that he had contracted leprosy. When Ram Bahadur Bista, the physiotherapist, confirmed that there was diminished sensation over the distribution of his thickened right ulnar nerve, Ramesh was shattered. Anaesthetic fingers on a trapeze artist swinging to catch swaying ropes at incredible heights with no safety net below, is a disaster waiting to happen. In his case he had no option - if their parents did not swing, his kids would starve.

We discussed the care of anaesthetic limbs, and I knew from the look in his glazed eyes that he was miles away. We started him on treatment and he came back to see me a couple of times with his wife when the circus was in town. A devoted wife with no signs of the disease, she assured me that she would never leave Ramesh. The visits stopped when the circus left town and I often wondered how they could have any continuity or follow-ups when they resumed their nomadic lifestyle. I will never forget the look of defeat I saw in his eyes when we confirmed his diagnosis. Confirming a patient's fears is the worst part of being a doctor. Sometimes you wish you could tell them something different to allay their fears. Ramesh had come to me with hope, wanting to hear that he did not have leprosy. He wanted me to make his fears go away, possibly in his mother tongue, Malayalam, when on Nepali soil. All I did was turn his life upside down before he moved out of my life. I never saw Ramesh again, but I have never forgotten him or the sadness in his eyes.

Patan skin clinic

Nirmala and James Nakami, our senior paramedics, were the backbone of every leprosy clinic in Anandaban and the UMN Shantha Bhavan Hospital in Patan. Patients were treated as outpatients in Shanta Bhavan once a week; only those who needed admission were brought back to Anandaban in the hospital Land Rovers.

The entire database of patients, bundles of yellow dog-eared medical record cards packed in two dusty steel trunks, travelled to and from Patan in the clinic Land Rover. The cards were catalogued and coded in a language only the Nakamis could decipher. The clinic would have ground to a halt without them. They were part of the pioneer staff that had been with Anandaban from its inception and knew every patient by face and name. It only took an old patient to step into the clinic and smile at them for James, or Massa as he was affectionately known, and Nirmala to fish out their medical records from their steel trunks and register them. Doctors would come and go, nurses would come and go, staff would come and go - ultimately it was the faithful paramedical team headed by Massa James that held the patients together with consistency and dedication. Theirs were the faces that the patients sought out when they walked into the OPD.

Bir hospital

When we joined Anandaban Hospital, I went to work at Bir Hospital in Kathmandu in the mornings with Dr Savitri Gurung, the HOD of the Ob/Gyn unit, to keep my Ob/Gyn skills alive. The kids and I would travel to Kathmandu in the school vehicle and I would get dropped off at Bir Hospital and picked up when the kids finished school in the afternoon. On my return to Anandaban, I would start my ward rounds and ulcer care. As the general work in Anandaban increased and my training in reconstructive surgery became a priority, I stopped going to Bir Hospital and concentrated on my work in Anandaban.

Training in reconstructive surgery

I found reconstructive surgery fascinating when a functioning tendon inserted into a paralysed muscle would restore lost movement and function. The restoration of function was as exciting and rewarding as was the joy on the patients' faces when they saw the restorative changes of surgery. I was fortunate to have been trained by several stalwarts from India and overseas. Nepal being a popular destination, we had a steady stream of visiting consultants who spent months with us on their extended WHO postings in Anandaban. Each had their particular brand of clinical skills, compassion, and treatment modalities. No matter where they came from, one constant connected all the dots in my training. The patient's needs came first.

I was sent to the Naini Leprosy Hospital near Allahabad to be trained by Dr Vijaykumar for a while. A highly skilled and gifted reconstructive surgeon, he and his lovely wife Sheeba kept me in their home and looked after me with a generosity of spirit that left me humbled. Every night they did a comic song and dance routine that had us in splits when we said goodnight. Armed with two scrawny sticks, the good doctor and his wife would conduct a dramatic and theatrical search of my room. Only when they were assured that no convict from the Allahabad Jail nearby was hiding under my bed would they allow me to retire for the night. We laugh about it even today!

Dr Saro Thangaraj, a reconstructive surgeon from India, a constant source of encouragement, is someone I remember fondly with gratitude. She used to visit Anandaban regularly to upgrade my surgical training. She was a kind and patient teacher, and the OT staff—Ruchal, Maila, Bachuram, Nobu and I—loved her and looked forward to her visits.

She taught me volumes in the hospital on the ulcer rounds. She would watch as I cleaned and dressed the ulcers after debridement offering valuable tips. On her return to Delhi, she would enquire about the status of the ulcer, never forgetting the patient's name. No detail was ever too unimportant for her. She never stayed at the guest house. She always stayed with us and took part in all the capers in the household. I always felt that a favourite aunt, who incidentally was a surgeon too, had come to visit. We swapped stories of parenting and shared all the humorous episodes of our kids. Rekha and Anish, were very happy to have her as an ally and as a buffer against discipline whenever she stayed with us. As a family we were so isolated and far from home and all things familiar that we were absolutely delighted when she stayed with us. In and out of our kitchen, she was always appreciative of anything I cooked, even if some were unmitigated disasters. She taught me many recipes and kitchen hacks that always still remind me of her.

When she unpacked, in addition to all the thoughtful presents she brought us, she would inevitably have something for the house - something she had noted was missing on a previous visit. Without a word she would bring it out for me because she knew some things were difficult to come by in Kathmandu. When the surgical cases were done and dusted, we used to go shopping together with a great deal of giggling and fun. She adored her kids—Harry, Sunil, and Sheila—and her shopping revolved around them. On one of her visits her suitcase broke and needed replacement. We went searching for a sturdy suitcase that would bear her punishing travel schedule. At the Samsonite shop, the poster on the wall claimed that *Even if the plane crashes, your suitcase will be intact*. Wasting no time, the salesperson took off from where the poster ended. A sucker for catchy adverts and not wanting to be left out, I joined the salesman and tried to convince her to buy the Samsonite. When Dr Saro laughed, her eyes would fill with tears that threatened to spill over. She laughed so much and so hard that the tears in her eyes spilled over her cheeks and she asked me, *Susie, if the plane crashes, who cares about the suitcase?*

Dr AJ Selvapandian, our orthopaedics professor from CMC Vellore, who spent several months with us in Anandaban on multiple WHO assignments, trained me to do BK (Below

Knee) amputations confidently and on my own. Dr Ernest Fritschi conducted several workshops on the care of leprosy foot in Anandaban. He believed that conservative treatment under compassionate hands inevitably scored over mutilating surgery. An unforgettable teacher, I learned volumes when he stayed with us.

Dr Tom Hirayama from the Department of Plastic Surgery, Tokyo Women's Medical University, was sponsored by Dr Yo Yuasa of the Sasakawa Foundation to spend time with us in Anandaban. He taught me several customised, aesthetic, and reconstructive procedures for leprosy faces. Dr Yuasa was the medical superintendent of the Anandaban Leprosy Hospital before he joined the Sasakawa Foundation as its medical director. He never forgot Anandaban and he always had a soft corner for it. No request from Anandaban for growth or research was ever too small or turned down. Thanks to Dr Yuasa and Dr Hirayama, several aesthetic reconstructive procedures, which had until then been out of reach for leprosy patients, were performed at Anandaban. The facelifts knocked years off patients and postoperatively left many of them unrecognisable even to themselves. Restoration of lost looks with lost function in a scarred human being can be quite electrifying.

Reconstructive surgery at Anandaban

Soon I was doing tendon transfers, BK amputations, and cosmetic surgery to the face, under local and spinal anaesthesia. Maila, Ruchal, Bachuram, Nobu Miyazaki a staff nurse from Japan and I formed the surgical team in Anandaban. They were all more experienced than I was, having worked with several experienced surgeons before me. I learned a great deal from them not only about leprosy and reconstructive surgery but also about loving, living, and giving. I will never forget their simplicity, goodness, and kindness to me. I would never have survived in Anandaban doing all the complicated surgeries if I had not been blessed to have them working alongside me.

Though Ruchal was trained to craft artificial limbs, he could do almost anything because he was committed, smart, and a quick learner who absorbed everything around him quietly and efficiently with his own brand of dignity. Maila, the genie in the operation theatre, and young Bachuram, his assistant, set the stage for a well-orchestrated performance each time, every time. The operation theatre never needed artificial light as two of its four walls were large glass windows that let in natural light. We would start theatre days with prayers, on our knees on the theatre floor, and ask the Almighty to take over. A film crew lead by Mike Johnston came from England to do a series for Channel 4. Seeing us in action, he said that we reminded him of an orchestra, where everyone knew their part well, and coordinated with the other with minimum wastage of time and effort. I never had to ask for anything during surgery. I merely put out my hand, and Maila would put the correct instrument. If I groped or fumbled, he would gently prise it out of my hand and replace it with something more appropriate. I would ask Maila and Ruchal unashamedly for advice whenever I needed it and for approval at every step of the operation. They were my right hand and my left, and we did everything from tendon transfers to facelifts to amputations. I will never forget their unstinting support or their kindness and generosity of spirit as they guided me through my surgical tenure at Anandaban.

Post-op physiotherapy

For reconstructive surgery in leprosy to have a successful outcome, it is crucial that the physiotherapists handling the cases after the plaster casts are removed are skilled, patient, and empathetic. Retraining of rerouted muscles and the return of function depends entirely on them, especially when dealing with the very young and the elderly. We were lucky to have Ram Bahadur Bista as a physiotherapist as he always gave it his best shot.

When the Post-op plaster casts had to be removed, the younger kids used to be terrified when Bista brought the noisy rotating electric blades near them. Sitting on a bench, I used to have them on my lap facing me with their arms wrapped tightly around me. They would bury their faces into my neck and keep their eyes closed as we hugged each other. Truth be told, I would be just as terrified as they of the outcome of the tendon transfer operations. So much could have gone horribly wrong but did not - so many miracles that left me amazed at God's grace and mercy.

Mycobacterial research laboratories

Meanwhile, Sam cleaned out one of the wards to start the Mycobacterial Research Laboratories. Wards that house leprosy patients for years are full of nooks and crannies where patients hide everything from pets to hooch and vegetables. Chillies, hung out to dry, would be strung across the ward like bunting alongside their laundry. After he relocated the patients, he spent weeks scrubbing and fumigating the space before painting it afresh to secure a sterile environment. Plodding on, he set up a research laboratory from scratch to do in vivo studies in thymectomised mice in leprosy. No mean task given the challenges in terrain, travel, and communication. Soon drug trials and immunotherapy were underway, transforming Anandaban from a sleepy leprosy home nestling in a pine forest in the Himalayas into a research centre on the international map.

Sam used to travel overseas and return with cages of nude mice that did not impress anyone. *All mice are nude for goodness sake,* joked the hospital staff. The staff at the airport christened him the *musa doctor*: the *mouse doctor* who travelled overseas to bring mice. One day, Nara Bahadur, one of the drivers who used to drive Sam to and from the airport, asked me in bewilderment why the otherwise apparently normal doctor-sahib, needed to travel out of the country to collect mice. He claimed that he had better-looking mice in his house that would cost next to nothing!

Sam chose to work in leprosy and HIV/AIDS all his life. Later, when he joined as the head of the newly instituted Department of Experimental Medicine at Tamil Nadu MGR Medical University in Chennai, his experience in leprosy in Nepal and Bhutan stood him in good stead for the twenty years he served there in the field of HIV/AIDS. His primary interest was in the area of mother-to-child transmission of the disease, which earned him the nickname *Father-of-the-mother-to-child-transmission-programme-of-HIV/AIDS.*

Well read, well informed and given his phenomenal knowledge of current affairs Sam is a great conversationalist. He can talk to anyone dustman or duke, stranger or friend, about anything from health-related issues to politics. Anything really. Topics mere mortals would balk at, leave alone discuss! Whenever and wherever he could, be it a social gathering at home or at a friend's place; on a plane or a train; at a petrol bunk, supermarket, or barber shop; in a men's toilet; or during a coffee break at church, he would patiently explain the disease to anyone willing to listen. Invariably, a curious audience would gravitate around him. The kids and I would watch him in fear and trepidation as he answered strangers' questions extremely professionally, especially those on *socially taboo* topics. In addition to his research in the then relatively unknown disease, Sam spent a great deal of time and effort organising workshops and conferences to educate communities, medical students, doctors, and other health workers on HIV/AIDS. He believed that disseminating knowledge and training was the only way forward. Dispelling their fears would make them better equipped to handle the HIV/AIDS epidemic that appeared in 1983 with India as an epicentre in southern Asia.

Our kids as teenagers used to be exasperated and acutely embarrassed when their Dad waxed eloquent about HIV/AIDS/condoms/MSM (men who have sex with men)/CSW (commercial sex workers), and so on, at parties, especially when their friends were present. *This Daddy is too much, Mummy*, they would complain bitterly, *You can't take him anywhere!* Only when they became adults did they begin to appreciate and respect his commitment to his work. It was never a job with Sam. It was always a crusade against two diseases similar in so many ways and yet so very different in so many other ways. Dreaded diseases shrouded with misconception, stigma, and ostracism.

The last outcasts

June Goodfield, the author of the book *From the Face of the Earth*, wrote about five diseases: kuru, hepatitis B, schistosomiasis, leprosy, and smallpox, the miracle of the century as far as eradication is concerned. The chapter on leprosy featured life in the Anandaban Hospital.

When Mike Johnstone, the leader of the BBC film crew, came out on a pilot trip, I was in the theatre doing a below-knee amputation. *Do you mind if I stay and watch?* he asked, as he stepped into a world very different from his. He had never visited a leprosy hospital before. He came for a day and stayed for several days, mesmerised by all that he saw around him. He spent time with the paramedics and nurses who walked him through the wards and field trips, translating his interviews with the patients.

The shutter of his camera never stopped clicking as he took pictures of Anandaban and the patients who filled the wards. Later, David Colliston arrived with his film crew and unending reels of film to shoot the documentary, *The Last Outcasts*. Moving patient accounts, including Ramesh's, the Malayalee trapeze artiste, and Shanta Maya's, the wife who was banished to the pigsty by her cruel husband, were portrayed.

Leprosy has broken up families down the centuries. What happened in earlier times continues to happen despite advances in healthcare, education, and awareness, with just a hint of change. Discrimination looms large and affects lives and livelihoods. *The Last Outcasts* was an attempt to dispel the fears and the cruel stigma surrounding the disease. The Mycobacterial Research Laboratories and the experiments with nude mice were showcased. Anandaban, despite all the odds of terrain and travel, had found a place in the world of research on leprosy.

When *The Last Outcasts* was aired, I was flown to Montreux, a quaint little Swiss town with squeaky-clean streets on the banks of the Lake Geneva at the foot of the Alps, to introduce the movie. It was an enchanting experience to wake up each morning in a quaint hotel room that looked out onto the tranquil lake and the snow-capped mountains. The theme of the hotel was the legend of William Tell. Every night, when I went back to my room, there would be fresh apples in a tray waiting for me. One of the apples would have an arrow running through it depicting the folklore of the German *Apfelschuss*: shooting an apple placed on a child's head to depict a feat of marksmanship with the crossbow. We were wined and dined like royalty and treated to the finest wine and gourmet cheese the size of a room while cuckoo clocks in all shapes and sizes harmoniously chimed away the time.

Seva Padak

In appreciation of his work in Nepal, Sam was awarded the Seva Padak by His Majesty the late King Birendra of Nepal at an investiture ceremony in the Narayanhiti Palace in Kathmandu. There was an animated debate about whether Sam should wear Nepali traditional dress for the ceremony or a suit. Sam chose to be comfortable and wore a suit.

When he reached the palace, he was put through a rehearsal. He had to hand over a one-rupee coin with his right hand to King Birendra in a symbolic gesture. Sam was so nervous he dropped the coin just as he was face-to-face with King Birendra. Mortified, he watched the coin roll away across the red carpet. Seeing his discomfiture, an amused King Birendra smiled and patted Sam on the shoulder and said, *It's ok, Doctor*. King Birendra then pinned the silver Seva Padak onto the lapel of his suit. Sam acknowledged it gratefully as a gesture from a monarch in appreciation of the teamwork of the devoted staff of the Anandaban Leprosy Hospital. *A leader is only as good as his team,* Sam always believed.

Years later, in Chennai, we saw the blood curdling pictures on TV of King Birendra's assassination together with other members of the royal family, and we wept to see the carnage. Princess Shanti Singh, the King's sister, another victim of the assassination, was a frequent visitor at the hospital as she was the patron for leprosy work in Nepal. I remember the numerous occasions when I took her around the hospital to bring her up to speed on the new projects completed and underway. These were real-life characters we had interacted with. We watched in disbelief as frame after frame showed pictures of the slain royal family and a nation's grief at the irreplaceable loss of a benevolent monarch and dynasty.

Prince Dhirendra, the King's younger brother, another

victim of the assassination, often travelled incognito around Nepal. One evening, as I was going home from work, I saw a car pull up at the steps that led to the hospital's main entrance. A young man in a printed T-shirt, jeans, and a pair of sneakers bounded up and asked if he could have a look around the hospital. We were used to visitors dropping in to see the place and encouraged these visits to minimise the stigma attached to a leprosy hospital. As Sam was away, I took him around and showed him the place. He seemed very interested in the patients and the facilities and chatted for a while with the patients, who seemed very happy to see him. Perhaps some of them had recognised him. I had absolutely no clue who he was until he got into the car to leave, when he turned to me rather cheekily and informed me that he was the King's youngest brother, HRH Prince Dhirendra!

We treasure the fond memories we have of HM King Birendra, HM Queen Aishwarya, HRH Princess Shanti, HRH Prince Dhirendra, and all the other members of the royal family of Nepal. We especially remember King Birendra as a kind and benevolent monarch who cared deeply for his people. RIP.

General clinics at Anandaban

As general hospitals in Kathmandu were reluctant to accept leprosy patients, we had to take care of all our leprosy patients' medical and surgical needs. In order to reduce the stigma associated with a leprosy hospital, we introduced a general OPD in Nepal for the surrounding villages just as we had in Bhutan.

Initially, people came only in emergencies, when circumstances made the trek to a hospital in Kathmandu difficult. With time, as word spread, people came from villages far and near to attend the general OPD forgetting that they were making tracks to a leprosy hospital. No two days in the general OPD of Anandaban were the same, and there was no way of predicting who or what would arrive at the OPD steps, either walking or carried in a basket. In addition to infections, diarrhoeas, and other common ailments, we saw some unusual cases that baffled us. Some nights we slept with no interruptions at all, and some nights we were up all night. We saw bizarre cases like animal mauls and bites while curious cases of poisoning were a regular feature. The injuries we had to deal with could have been the result of anything from domestic abuse and drunken brawls to attempted suicides.

I remember a tragic case when an eight-month-old child was brought to the OPD with a history of snakebite on her right hand forty-eight hours prior to being seen in OPD. The grandmother had walked for many miles carrying the child on her hip. To stop the spread of the venom in the child's body, she had tied a tight rubber tube as a makeshift tourniquet on the right upper arm about four inches above the elbow. I could have cried when I saw the child. The right arm was swollen and cyanosed a mottled blue, below the tourniquet. Strangely, the child was not in any discomfort, nor was she crying in pain. We referred them to an orthopaedic surgeon in Bir Hospital. Unfortunately, the limb could not be saved, and the baby lives her life as an amputee.

In another bizarre case, an apparently healthy postmenopausal woman walked into the OPD from a village a few miles away with a history of sudden onset of vaginal bleeding for four days. The painless and episodic vaginal bleeding conjured up several sinister possibilities in my mind. A speculum examination revealed a couple of stowaways in her vagina. On questioning, she said that she had gone to visit her daughter in the next village and had taken a shortcut through the river that flowed in front of her house. While wading across the river, she had unwittingly picked up a couple of leeches that had attached themselves to her vagina. Turgid and tenacious, one was hanging to the posterior vaginal wall, close to the introitus, and the other hung higher up in the posterior fornix of the vagina. Plucking them out with a pair of forceps was not an option as I had no clue about the leeches' mouthparts or sucker apparatus, but common sense told me that plucking them out could cause tissue damage and uncontrolled bleeding. So, I did the next best thing: I used a xylocaine spray to stun them so that they would loosen their hold on the vaginal mucosa. After a few minutes, the leeches relaxed their vice-like grip and fell off. A saline douche irrigated her vagina, and a vaginal pack for an hour prevented any further bleeding. Leeches in the vagina never figured in any of my textbooks in college. Common sense was something we learnt to rely on, especially when all else failed.

Toxicology in the Himalayas
Cases of poisoning, each one more bizarre than the other, appeared every month in the OPD. There were no chapters in toxicology textbooks for the poisonous and noxious substances we came across in Bhutan and Nepal.

Sometimes the patients jumped off the bed with the metal retractor in their mouths halfway through the stomach wash and ran down the hill with the staff chasing them shouting, *Come back... Come back, the metal gag is still in your mouth!* One Sunday afternoon, just before lunch, Krishna the ward boy came charging down the hill to tell me that a new bride had been brought to the hospital. He was so distressed that he could not get the words out properly. He gasped and spluttered that she had attempted to commit suicide after a fight with her mother-in-law. Apparently, these fights were the order of the day in their home in the valley below. In a fit of rage, she broke the new red glass bangles that were a wedding gift from her husband, ground them between two layers of her sari, and swallowed them.

A stomach wash was definitely out of the question as it could do more harm than good. Spicules of glass chasing each other down the mucous lining of her GI tract was not a good idea. A practical option was to feed her masses of soft-boiled starchy rice and wait. And pray. We cleaned her mouth and checked for any major cuts. Assured that they were merely superficial lacerations, we started the IV drip and fed her with plain soft-boiled rice made into bite-size boluses. The staff sat with her for twenty-four hours, examining every stool she passed into a bedpan while keeping a close watch on her pulse and blood pressure and checking for signs of tenderness or guarding of the abdomen. Mercifully, she survived and returned with her mother-in-law a year later to deliver a baby. All's well that ends well apparently!

On payday, labourers would get drunk and eat poisonous berries in their inebriated state. These berries though not lethal, could trigger a nasty gastroenteritis leaving the men dangerously dehydrated and needing intravenous infusions. My broken Hindi, which worsened in highly stressful conditions, did not help much in medical emergencies. Since I had not studied Hindi as a second language in Singapore, I had to make do with what I had picked up from the Hindi movies I watched on borrowed DVDs, virtually the only entertainment we had in Anandaban. My curse words would, I am sure, have passed muster, but I gather my grammar was atrocious, and I know I often mixed-up words. Once when I was struggling to put the mouth gag in place for a stomach wash, I believe I turned to the patient impatiently and asked him how much he had drunk. *Kithna pishap peekay aaya*? Only when the staff burst out laughing did I realise that I had goofed. I had asked him how much urine he had drunk when I had meant to ask him how much liquor he had drunk. I had said *pishap* for *sharab*. Of course, I never heard the end of this faux pas, which I understand is still repeated in Anandaban.

In Hindi, there is a gender for everything and every object. I could never get it right. Nor did I get the pronouns *Thou* and *You* right. I would address the elderly with a disrespectful *You* and the K9 with an incongruous *Thou*. The kindly patients and staff learnt to live with my Hindi and forgave my every grammatical mistake.

The worst landslide of the century

While we were in Nepal, we witnessed one of the most tragic disasters of nature. The oldest man in the village, who had lived to a hundred, said that he had never seen such devastation in all his years. When we woke up that morning, we had no idea of the horrors that lay ahead. The morning seemed no different. The children tumbled out of bed, squabbled through breakfast, got dressed, and left for school, happy that Sam was going with them to Kathmandu in the school van. If their Dad travelled with them on the school trip for his work in Kathmandu, they knew that they would end up with all sorts of treats on their way home.

I waved them goodbye and went up to the hospital to start my work. It was the week before the harvest festival Dasara, and Nepal wore a festive look for this annual thanksgiving. This was a time to relax before winter set in. This was the time of the year when families headed home for the annual holidays and several days of merrymaking. New clothes would be bought and the girls would have new bangles to match the new red ribbons in their hair. Goats would be cut and local hooch would flow as families met and children went home to visit their parents. The roads would be busy with people travelling up and down as people flocked home.

After the ward rounds, we went into the operation theatre. The first case on the list was a foot drop, and we started the tendon transfer under spinal anaesthesia. Looking out through the glass windows of the theatre, I noticed that it had started raining, and before I knew it, turned into a never-ending torrential downpour. Suturing the tendon, I wondered if I had closed the windows at home. When it rained, we always got the rain in if we left the windows open. A few minutes later, the door of the theatre opened, and the manager, Pradeep Failbus, and Chandra Thapa, from the office, stuck their heads in to tell us that floods in Lele, the village on the hill above Anandaban, had caused a landslide.

Before this disturbing bit of information could sink in, Bachuram came charging in, visibly agitated, to report that the village below us, Chapagaon, was also flooded with a devastating landslide. Men and livestock had been swept down the river with the tide.

My blood ran cold. This was a nightmare that everyone worried about in Nepal. Ruthless deforestation denuded mountains that moved at the slightest provocation. This was the time of the year when both Lele and Chapagaon would be packed with shoppers from the local villages. There was no way anyone could have taken a headcount of the casualties.

I have no idea how we managed to finish the operation despite all the distractions, the frantic interruptions, and the disturbing news updates. Tearing off my gloves, I ran all the way down to a wet, noisy and crowded OPD to a visual that took my breath away. Pradeep had, with characteristic efficiency, rallied the staff to give first aid. Many of the children and adults that rescue teams had pulled out of the water were screaming in pain and terror, and strangers cuddled infants close to the warmth of their hearts. Terrified people huddled in groups against the whitewashed wall of the OPD. Some needed sutures. Some needed X-rays. Some just needed a plain white sheet to cover their lifeless bodies. The air was beginning to smell damp and dank. The staff were absolutely wonderful. Unasked, they ran down to their homes and brought dry, warm clothes, blankets, and food. Everyone pitched in to do whatever was needed to the best of their ability.

The road to Chapagaon was blocked, and Land Rover transfers to the bigger hospitals in Kathmandu were not an option. *Sam and the kids will never get through*, I thought to myself in an unguarded moment of panic. Reassured that Sam was with the kids, I pushed panic out of the way and got through the rest of the day and all the challenges the landslide and floods served up at the Anandaban hospital, which was ill-equipped to handle a disaster of this magnitude. By evening, the rain had stopped though the sky remained a sombre and menacing curtain. The casualties from the OPD were accommodated in the wards. Some of the kids whose parents never showed up went to their relatives' homes as orphans. Parents who had lost their own kids adopted kids who had lost their parents and home. Indeed, humanity shone through in the hour of need. Sam and the kids traipsed in wet, cold, and hungry late in the evening having walked back all the way from Chapagaon.

Meanwhile, scavengers were retrieving what they could from the riverbanks. One person's misfortune is instant wealth for another in a catastrophe and profiteering is extremely common in calamities of this magnitude. The goldsmith in Lele lost his life and his shop. A safe stacked with money and all the jewellery that villagers had pawned in times of financial trouble floated down the river and was never recovered. Whether it sank with its contents to lodge forever in the riverbed or whether it changed the tide and fortunes of mere mortals, one will never know. Among the injured was a family of four, a father, a mother, and their two children, with extensive second-degree burns. They had been sitting for a meal at their wooden dining table when lightning struck.

The survivors said that there were at least fifty people having tea at a local tea shop. One minute they were all laughing and joking. The next minute they were washed away to a premature death. One minute, life was sailing along merrily, and the next minute it was a catastrophe. A tragedy leaving behind a trail of carnage. For weeks, the whole valley wore an uneasy calm as the stench from the decomposing bodies in the riverbed pervaded the air. The aftermath of the tragedy was palpable for a long time and the stream of the injured limping into the OPD continued over into the next few days and nights.

Dasara that year was a bleak and dismal affair as villagers continued to wait for missing relatives who never returned home.

Obstetrics in Nepal

Many women in rural Nepal in the early 1970s hesitated to have their babies in hospitals. There were many reasons for this. Firstly, they were on alien turf among strangers. Secondly, it was definitely more expensive than a home delivery. I discovered a third reason quite late into my stay in Nepal.

Once, during an annual hospital dinner to which the staff and their families were invited, I noticed that Sathya's wife was missing. Sathya the driver, as loyal as you make them, did the school run through the week and looked after Rekha and Anish like his own. When I asked him if she was unwell, he replied sheepishly that they had just had a baby a couple of days ago, and the placenta had not fallen off yet. That was the night I found out about an old Nepali custom.

For a host of cultural and religious reasons, Nepali mothers who delivered at home preferred not to cut the cord after the birth of the baby. The baby and the placenta remained attached. The placenta is kept in a mud pot alongside the infant until the cord shrivels up and drops off with the dry placenta. Only when the placenta and cord fell off was the woman considered cleansed and only then could she move out of the house. This may have been the reason why the incidence of cord sepsis and neonatal tetanus was low in Nepal because no unsterile instruments were ever used to cut the cord. This was also the third reason why many Nepali women hesitated to have their deliveries in hospitals. In the hospital, we cut the cord and throw the placenta into a bucket without a second glance unless we needed it to dress a non-healing ulcer in the ward.

When the deliveries were conducted at home, many women would have a prolonged third stage of labour with a retained placenta. Usually, the placenta is expelled within thirty minutes of the baby being delivered when the uterus contracts down. In retention of the placenta, this time is prolonged and often requires manual removal ideally under anaesthesia.

The most common cause for retention of the placenta is a full bladder. The bladder, the uterus, and the rectum are linked by slings that hold them in place. Dysfunction of one of these organs disturbs the normal functioning of the other. In the busyness of dilating her cervix and delivering the baby, the mother forgets to void her bladder which can cause retention of the placenta. This is potentially dangerous in home deliveries, especially as it increases the chances of postpartum haemorrhage and infection from all the manipulations that are tried, often unsuccessfully, to deliver the placenta manually.

I used to be called for house visits to nearby villages when a woman had a retained placenta. The first few times when they told me that the house was *just here*, I believed them and walked miles to reach the patient. Subsequently, I got smart and knew that the *just here* was anything but that. It could be several million steps on a pedometer I did not possess.

The first time I set off with the ward boys, the paramedics, and the patient's relatives, we drove to the nearest point on the road and then walked down a mud path that seemed to go on forever. Finally, we reached a three-storeyed house set in a wooded cluster. The ground floor housed the family's animals. The goats, the cows, and the dogs lay around perfectly at peace with the kids who played a short distance away. The family lived on the first floor, and the grain was stored on the second floor. To get to the top floor where the patient lay, I had to use the wooden ladder that leaned on the side. Did I just say leaned? No, correct that to, we had to climb up a wooden ladder that was screwed vertically into the building. I was inappropriately dressed in a sari. Definitely not the best attire to climb anything in. Kicking off my slippers, I nonchalantly tucked my sari between my legs and held on to the ladder and climbed as far as I could, with my eyes shut tight.

When I threatened to slip and fall all the way down, two of the ward boys pushed me up, very apologetically, from behind and two male relatives standing on the floor above, at the top of the ladder, took hold of my arms and pulled me up, and I landed unceremoniously with a thud on the mud floor. I was totally unprepared for the stench that hit me as I surfaced to take stock of my surroundings and the foul smell that made my head reel. I had landed in a dark and dank room that smelled of stale blood, stale urine, and human excreta. Gagging, I got up, too frightened to put one foot in front of the other, not knowing what I would step into. My eyes had accommodated to the poor light by then, and in the far corner, I saw a low bed and a silhouette sleeping on it.

Gingerly, I inched closer and got the shock of my life. Lying on it was a woman, stark naked, covered with a sheet of flies hovering over her. Propped up against the bedstead, she was swatting the flies around her listlessly with a vacant stare. She looked tired and dehydrated. Between her legs, in a pool of clotted blood, lay something long and twisted that looked like an umbilical cord that had stopped pulsating. There was a dirty cloth ball with a broken wooden stick through it tied to the cord – probably additional reinforcement when they had tried to pull at the cord. There was no sign or cry of any baby in the room. The ward boys had climbed up and reached the room by then. They positioned her flat on the bed and brought her near the edge of the bed. On examination, her vitals appeared normal. Her bladder seemed distended and needed catheterisation. Ignoring the obviously unsterile conditions, I put on a pair of gloves and catheterised her, letting the urine collect into a plastic bag the ward boy held out. No sooner had we done that, I saw her wince as if she was having a contraction. I pushed the contracted uterus gently away from her suprapubic region with my left hand and wound the fingers of my right hand around the cord to give it a gentle tug. To my utter and unmitigated relief, it came out freely, bringing the placenta with it, followed by a surge of blood that squirted everywhere.

We sponged her down with some cotton, got her dressed and padded, bundled her up in blankets, and put her in a cloth sling stretcher, something like the ones the proverbial storks brought babies in. They lowered the sling stretcher down carefully, navigated by a crowd of spectators who had gathered below.

When she had safely reached the ground floor, the ward boys strung the cloth sling stretcher onto a pole they balanced on their shoulders as they marched forward with the patient lying in the makeshift stretcher. I then slid and slithered down the vertical ladder and landed on the same behind that had been pushed up the perpendicular wooden staircase barely an hour earlier. Dusting myself, I got up laughing, helping to ease a tense and awkward situation. Somewhere in the far distance, I heard a baby cry. The baby had been rescued after birth and taken down to the grandmother who was waiting below with open arms. On examination, the infant appeared to be fine and none the worse for wear. Mother and baby were in safe hands and were on their way to the Anandaban Leprosy Hospital. We settled her in the Land Rover and drove back to the hospital where the staff was waiting for us. The nursing team was brilliant and took complete charge. They wheeled the mother away, mopped her up, and sponged her down. They started a drip, added the antibiotics, checked the cord, cleaned the baby, and settled the exhausted mother and child in a warm bed with clean sheets and a hot meal. The staff at Anandaban were amazing. They stepped in when needed and followed their instinct and training, rising admirably to the occasion. We would have been utterly lost without them.

I was cross-eyed and weary when I reached home. Shedding everything outside the bathroom, I had the longest bath ever, rubbing off layers of grime and dirt before I crashed, wondering what Dr Paranjothy, Dr Kunders, or Dr Prabha, for that matter, would have to say about my first encounter with a retained placenta in Nepal. Sam listened carefully when I brought him up to speed with a blow-by-blow account.

And this is the lady who lived in high heels, hated using the stairs, and went from one floor to another in a lift, he chuckled as he threw back his head and laughed.

Anandaban revisited

Thirty-three years after we left Anandaban, I returned to Nepal. En route to Anandaban, I spent a nostalgic afternoon with James and Nirmala Nakami in Kathmandu. We had all aged, but it did not dim the happy memories of our kids, Rekha and Anish, and their kids, John and Jenny, the inseparable *awesome foursome*, and all the mischief they would get up to. We cried when we remembered the staff we had loved and lost: Ruchal, Maila, Sathya, Tek Bahadur, and Dharma. We remembered patients and anecdotes that transported us to an Anandaban of the 1980s. We knew that we would never meet again when we said an emotional goodbye. Massa passed away a few weeks later, but I was happy and grateful to have met them and reconnected after all these years.

I spent a pleasant evening with Barnabas and Kunti Neupane in Kathmandu. Barnabas was a mere boy when he worked with us. The grey-haired gentleman who smiled at me over the head of his grandson playing on his lap was a mature version of the young, dedicated, and sincere male nurse who ran tirelessly up and down the wards built on the slope of a hill caring for his patients. It was lovely to see him as a grandfather, retired and settled well in the city.

Barnabas Neupane and Jenny Nakami accompanied me in the taxi that took me to Anandaban. I met Maya, the ward aide who had worked with us all those years ago. Her home was on the slope we had to climb to reach the hospital. She had developed COPD as she aged, a pulmonary condition that kept her anchored to an oxygen cylinder. Maya died two weeks after I met her, and I was truly glad to have met her after all these years - glad that we had a chance to reconnect and share some precious memories of the kids.

She was not expecting me as I had appeared without any warning. She burst into tears when she recognised me and held my face in her hands. Crying and laughing, we reminisced about the good old days. She remembered Anish, *Baba* to the staff. Maya had kept three of his goats with hers for safekeeping. Every day after school, he would run down the hill to check on his goats and play with them. When they multiplied, he came charging back to tell us that he had become a grandfather and even had names for them, names Maya remembered. She remembered Rekha bringing Pappoo and Tiny the Lhasa Apsos home from Kathmandu as tiny puppies in two wicker baskets. We laughed as we remembered them escaping from their baskets and hiding while Rekha desperately searched high and low for them.

Tingling with anticipation, excited to revisit our old home, I jumped out of the car at the landing that led to the medical superintendent's house, the home we had lived in as a young family and raised our kids. I froze in my tracks, totally unprepared for what met my eyes. There was no house. Our precious home no longer existed. All I could see was a flat piece of land with just one familiar landmark, the pine tree with the decussating branches resembling a tuning fork that stood at the right-hand corner of the plot.

The house was gone.

The devastating earthquake that shook Nepal in 2015 had destroyed numerous buildings on the Anandaban Hill including the Medical Superintendent's house. Our old house had been razed to the ground to construct a new building. However, it did not stop the memories from cascading down in sharp vivid colours. The audio-visuals of two kids rushing home excited to share their news from school did not seem to need the house to come alive. *Mummy ghar-ma choh? Is Mummy at home?* they would ask whoever they met, as they tumbled down the steps. If I was in the hospital, they would throw down their bags and water bottles to run up the slope to the hospital to find me, bursting with news from school that they could not wait to share. *Mummy, you will never guess what happened…* was a favourite opening line. Precious bits of paper would be held up for approval as they jostled for attention. All their latest trophies of war, their cuts and bruises, would need to be inspected. A scraped knee, a broken nail, a chipped tooth, a torn dress, a broken pencil or rubber, all viewed and inspected before they ran off to have their milk and cookies. I do not remember them walking. They either skipped or ran. I do not think they knew how to walk. It did not matter that our home had been razed to the ground. My memories did not need brick and mortar. My precious memories were housed in my heart for eternity. As indeed were my memories of life in Anandaban. Tearing up, I turned and walked up the familiar steps that led up to the main hospital.

The patients evacuated from the wards were accommodated in makeshift tents on the playing ground, waiting for the new wards under construction. The old was making way for the new with the promise of a dramatic makeover. Many of the staff who had worked with us had either retired or passed away. Some who heard that I was visiting came up from their villages to meet me. The grey in their hair did not in any way dim the affection in their eyes and smiles.

The icing on the cake was a board that read **The Leprosy Mission Nepal,** something that Sam fantasised about when we worked there in the 80s. It took more than twenty years for TLM Nepal to be established in 2015 as an independent NGO working in partnership with TLM International and the Government of Nepal. The Anandaban Leprosy Hospital no longer needs to wait in a long queue with several other hospitals in another country for sanctions and permissions to expand and grow to meet its needs. Anandaban's needs are now completely addressed hands on by Nepal on home ground. Anandaban, cradled in prayer, has come into its own and stands as a place reflecting God's love and providing comprehensive care to the Leprosy patients of Nepal and their healthcare givers.

    I was returning to Anandaban after more than three decades. I had changed. Anandaban had changed. People had changed. Circumstances had changed. The world had changed. Why even my cup had overflowed and I was drinking from the saucer! Only one thing had not changed. Hanging on a branch of one of the pine trees of Anandaban, the Forest of Joy, was a piece of my heart that will always beat for all the patients we were privileged to have loved and served. The larger than life teachers who taught me valuable lessons that I dare not forget.

Thank you God!

Thank you

Dear God, for making it all happen with infinite grace, mercy, and blessings beyond belief

Mini Krishnan, The Bear would never have worn the swimsuit if not for you

Annammal Paatti, my dear grandmother for your unconditional love

Appachan and *Ammachy*, my beloved Dad and Mum for your tough love that equipped me for life

Sam, Rekha, Nitil, Anish, Vidhu, Ashish, and Rohan, my precious family, for your unstinting support

My Kodukulanji Kousins, my med school class of 1964, and all my dear friends for cheering me on

Malati Mukherjee and Team Words and Space, for rescuing me from drowning in my own words

Ivy Mary George and the St Margarets School Alumni who at short notice scoured the island for the school magazines of the 60s

Vijailakshmi Acharya, my dear friend for your invaluable advice

Vincent Moses Raja for your infinite patience

Chetan Acharya and Raji Srinivasan for restoring precious photographs and forgotten memories

Sashikala Asirvatham, for your meticulous finishing touches to The Bear

Renu Kaul Verma, V. Bhavani and Team Vitasta for risking a run with a rookie

Parish of Christ Church Singapore Website, Kapil Dev Neupane, Barnabas Neupane, Pradeep Failbus, Shantha & Bruce Duncan, George Mathew, Jacob Mathew, Saras Sinniah and Indra Pucknill for collage contributions

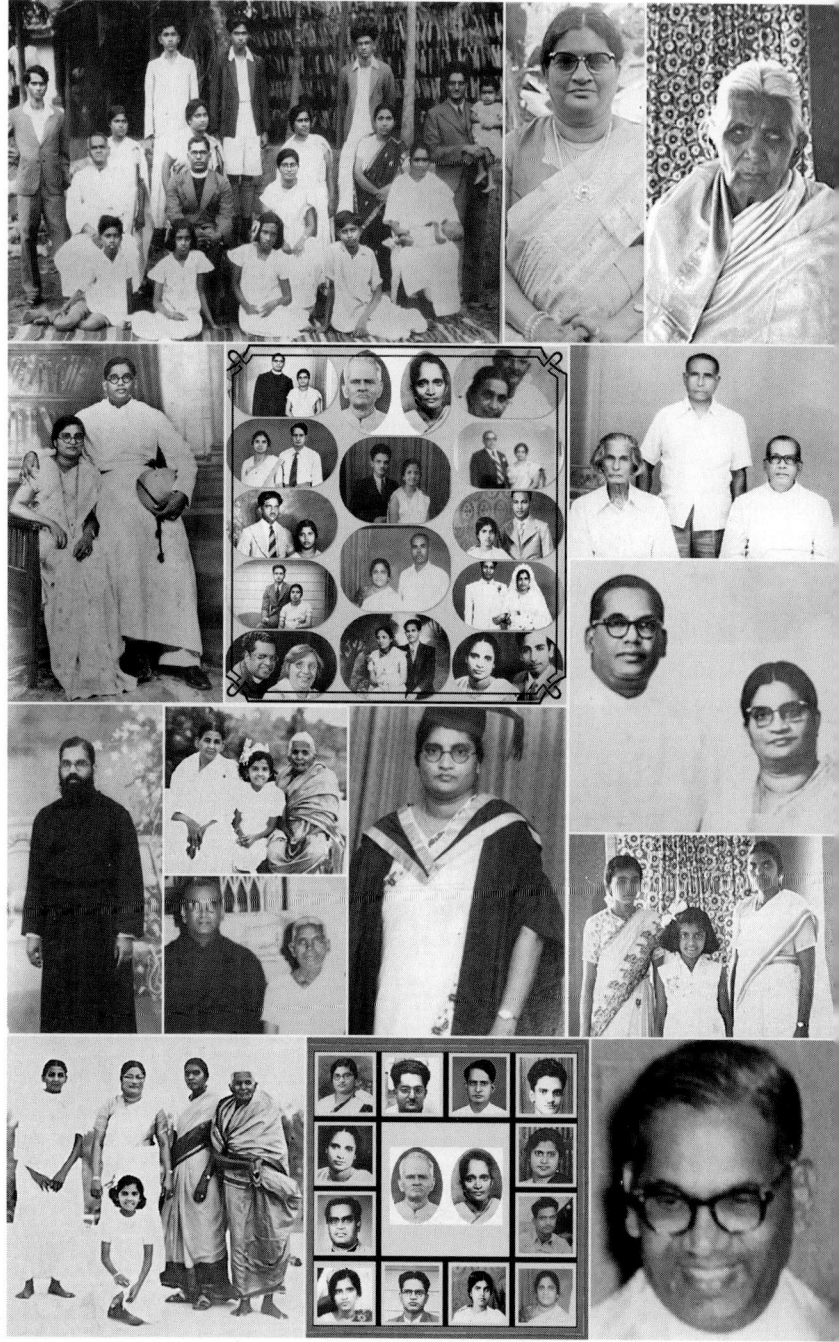

In the begining

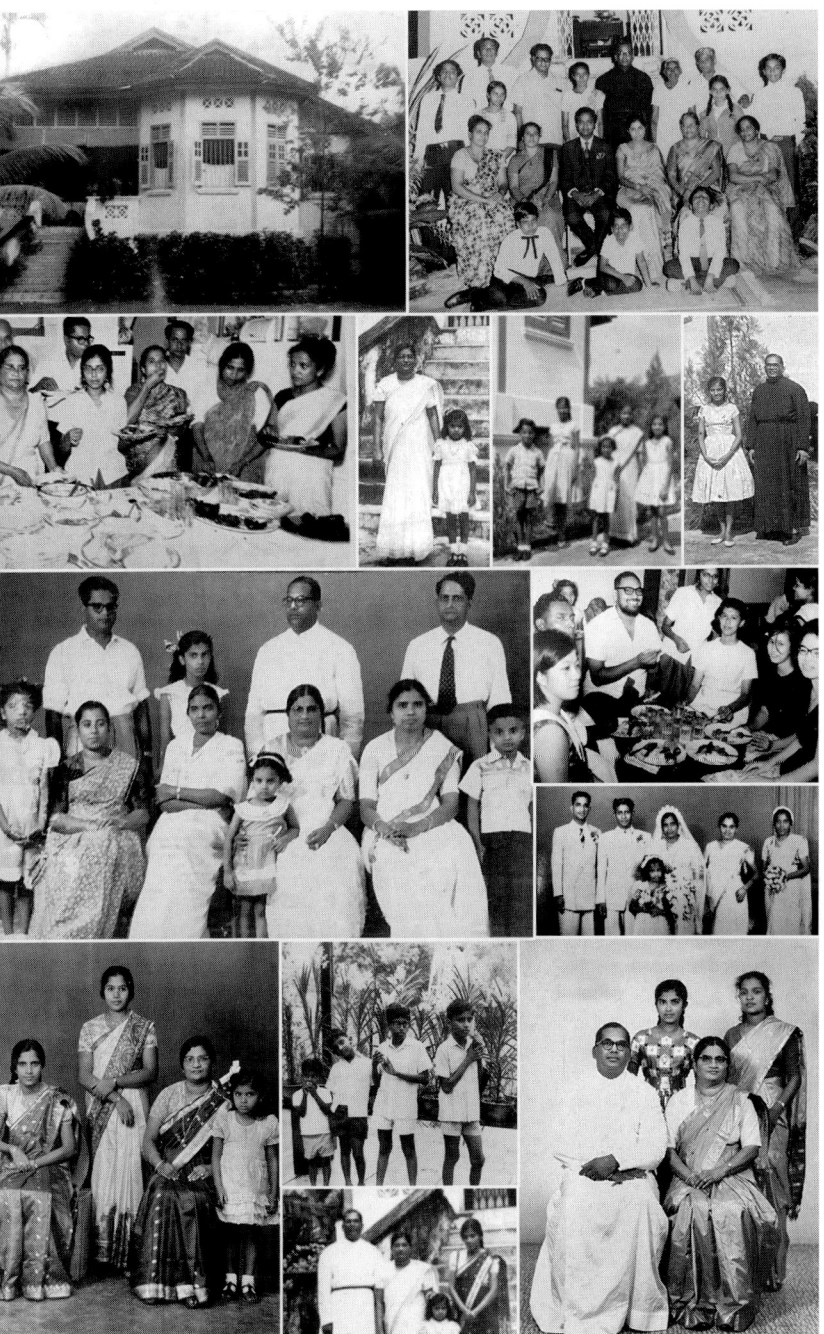

The Parsonage

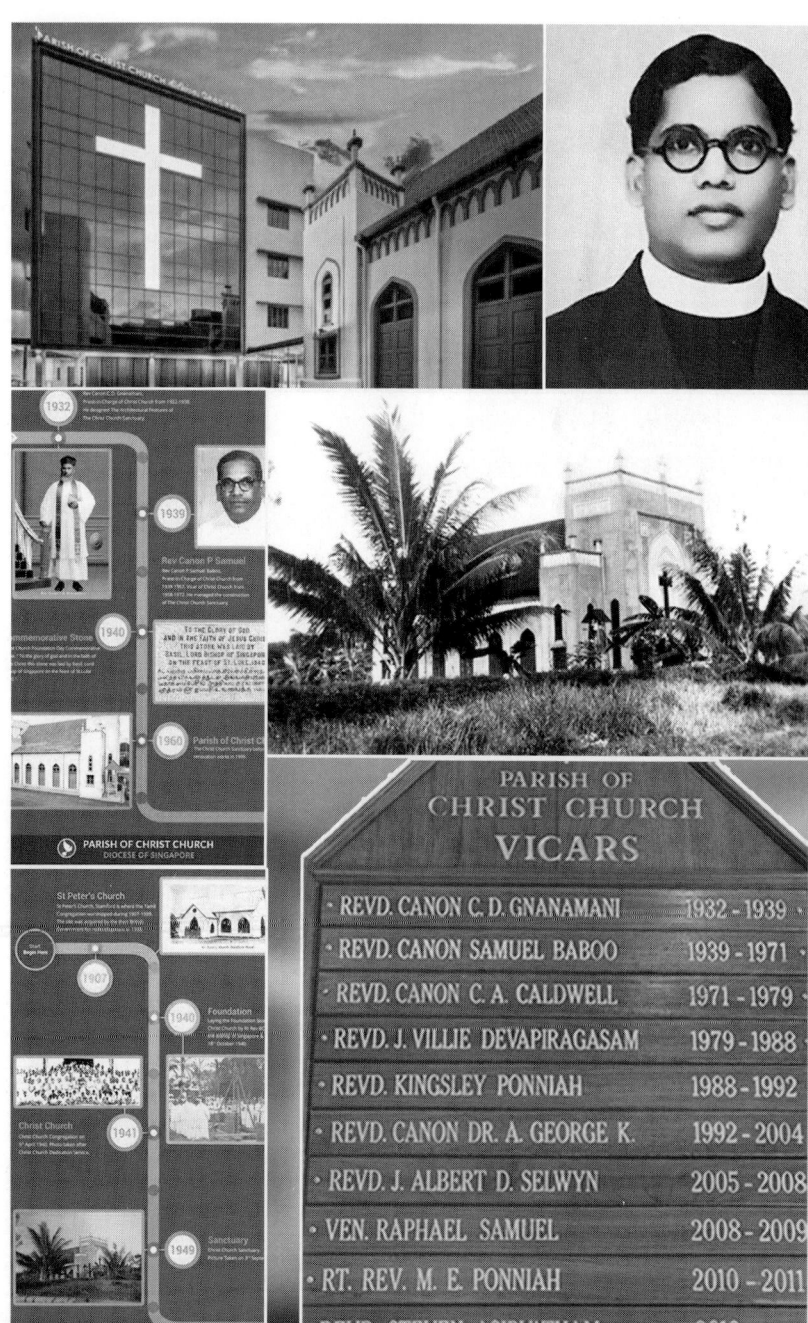

Christ Church Singapore

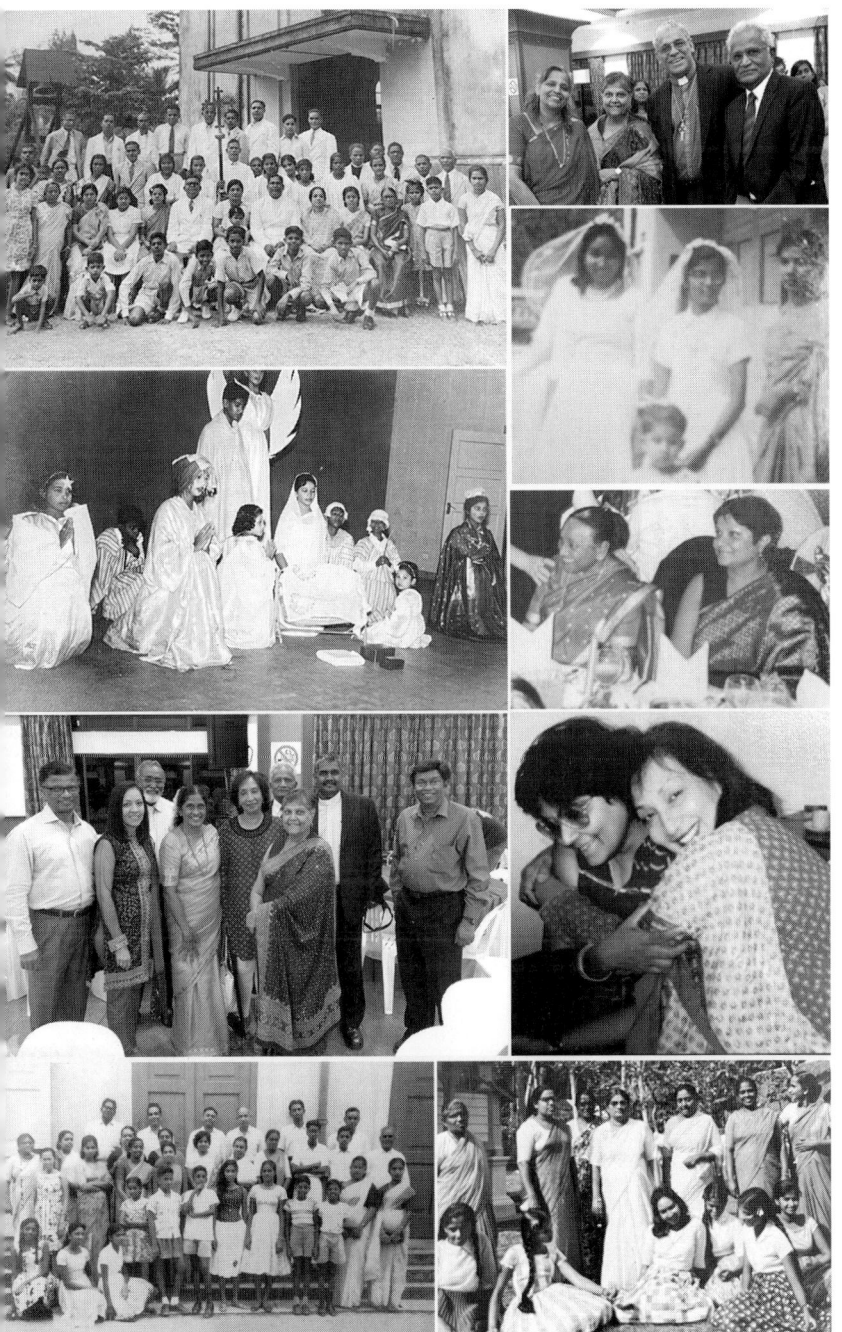

Christ Church Family

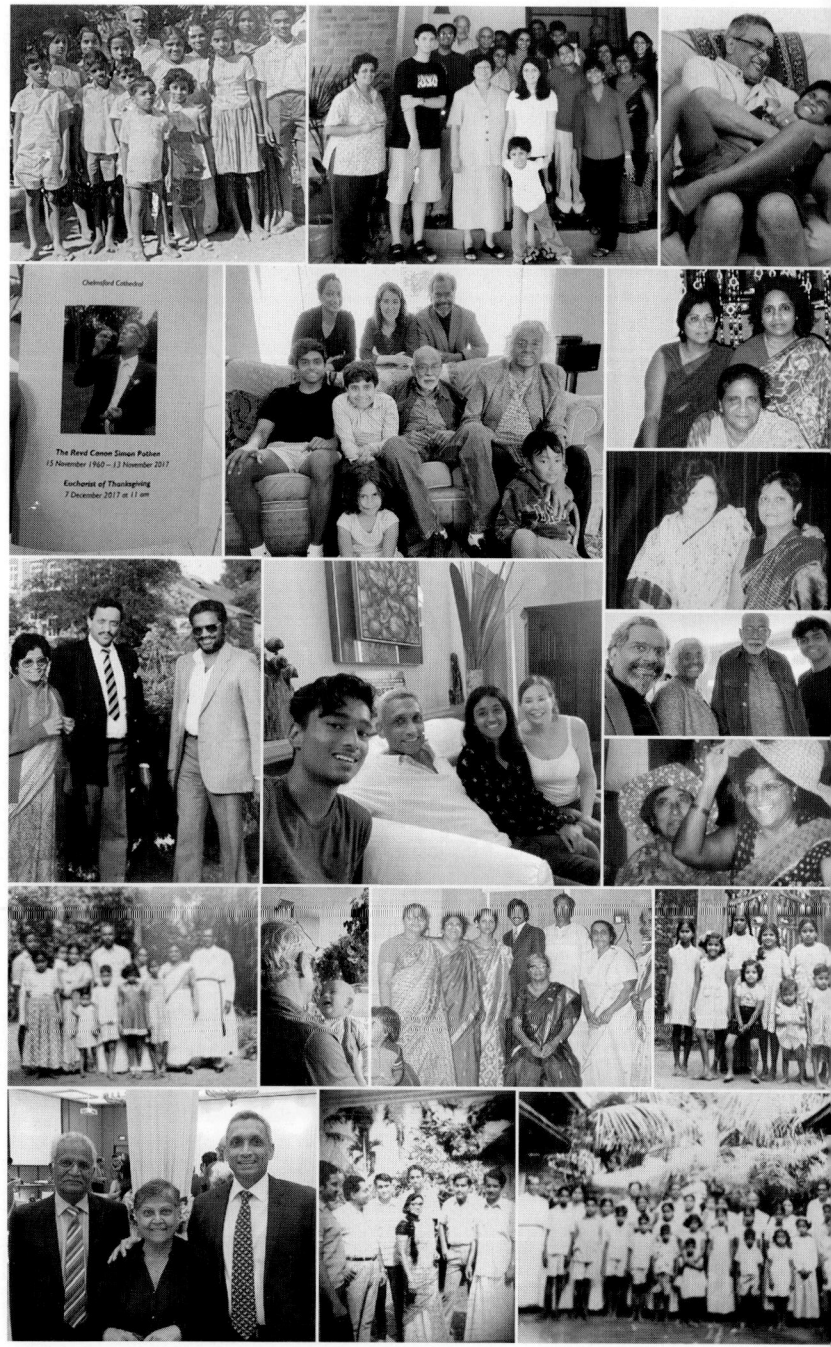

Kodukulanji Kousins 1

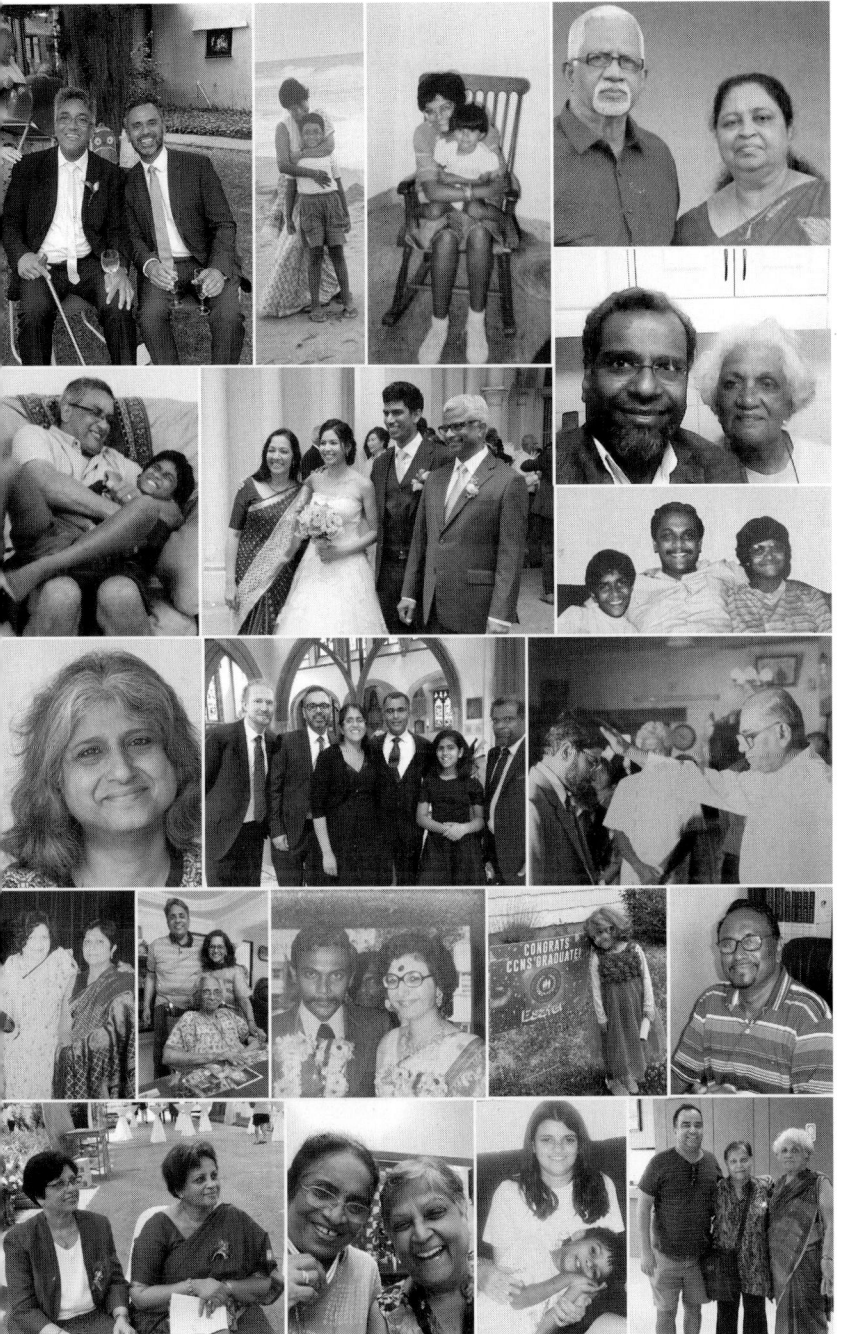

Kodukulanji Kousins 2

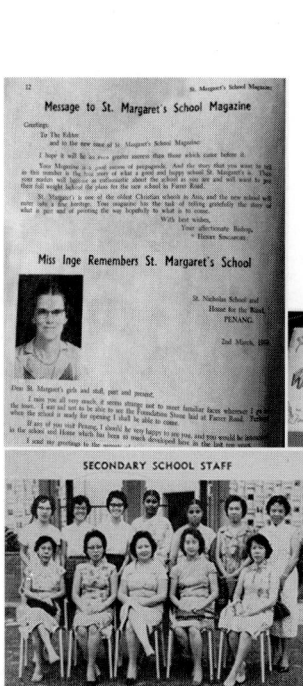
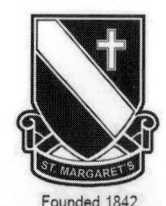
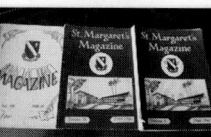
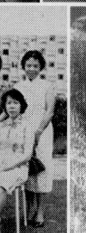
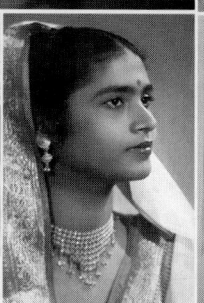
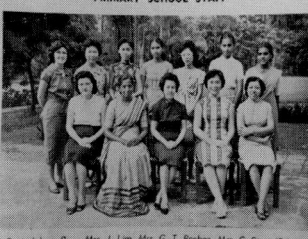
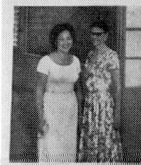
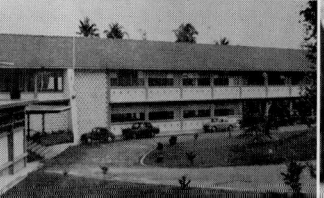
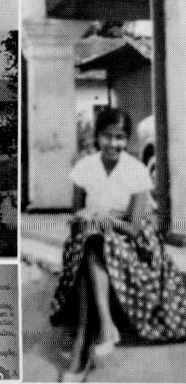
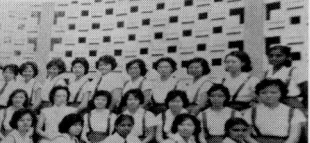
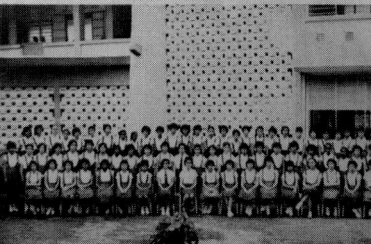

St Margarets Singapore

TRUTH CHARITY

STELLA MARIS COLLEGE

(AUTONOMOUS), CHENNAI - TAMILNADU

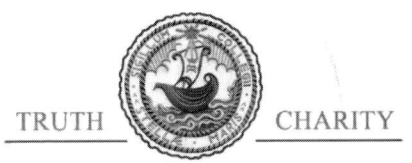

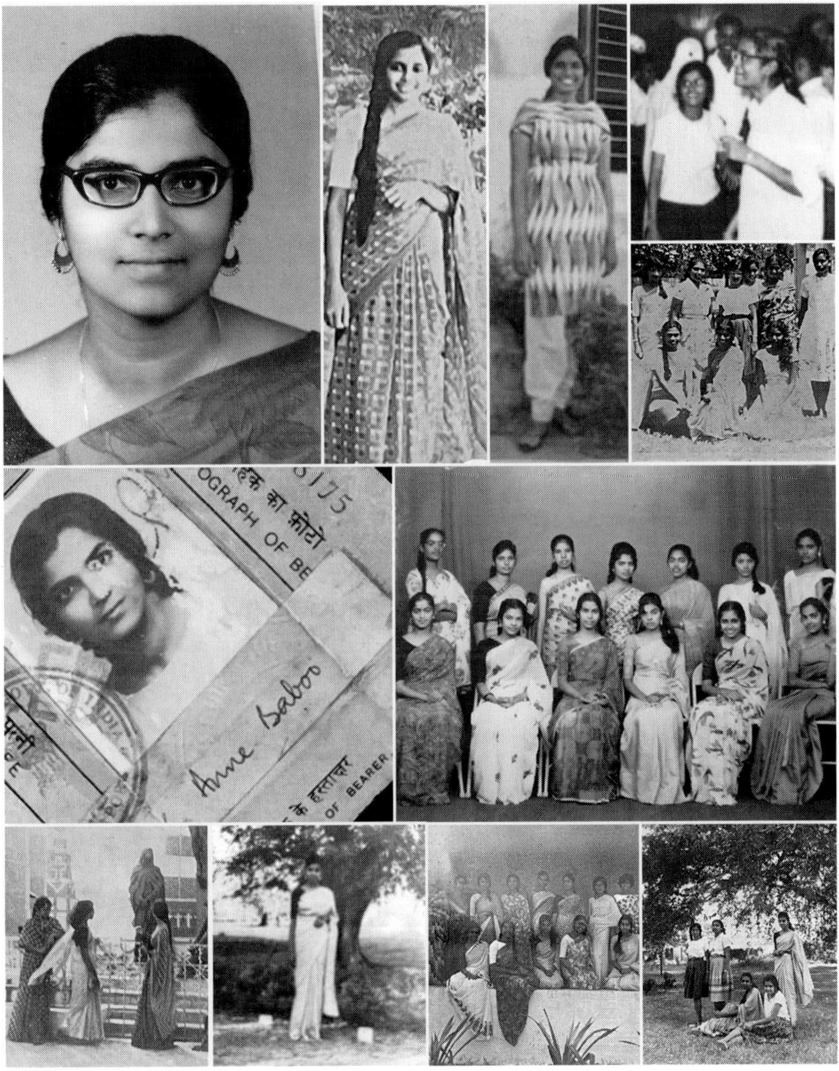

Stella Maris PU 7, Madras

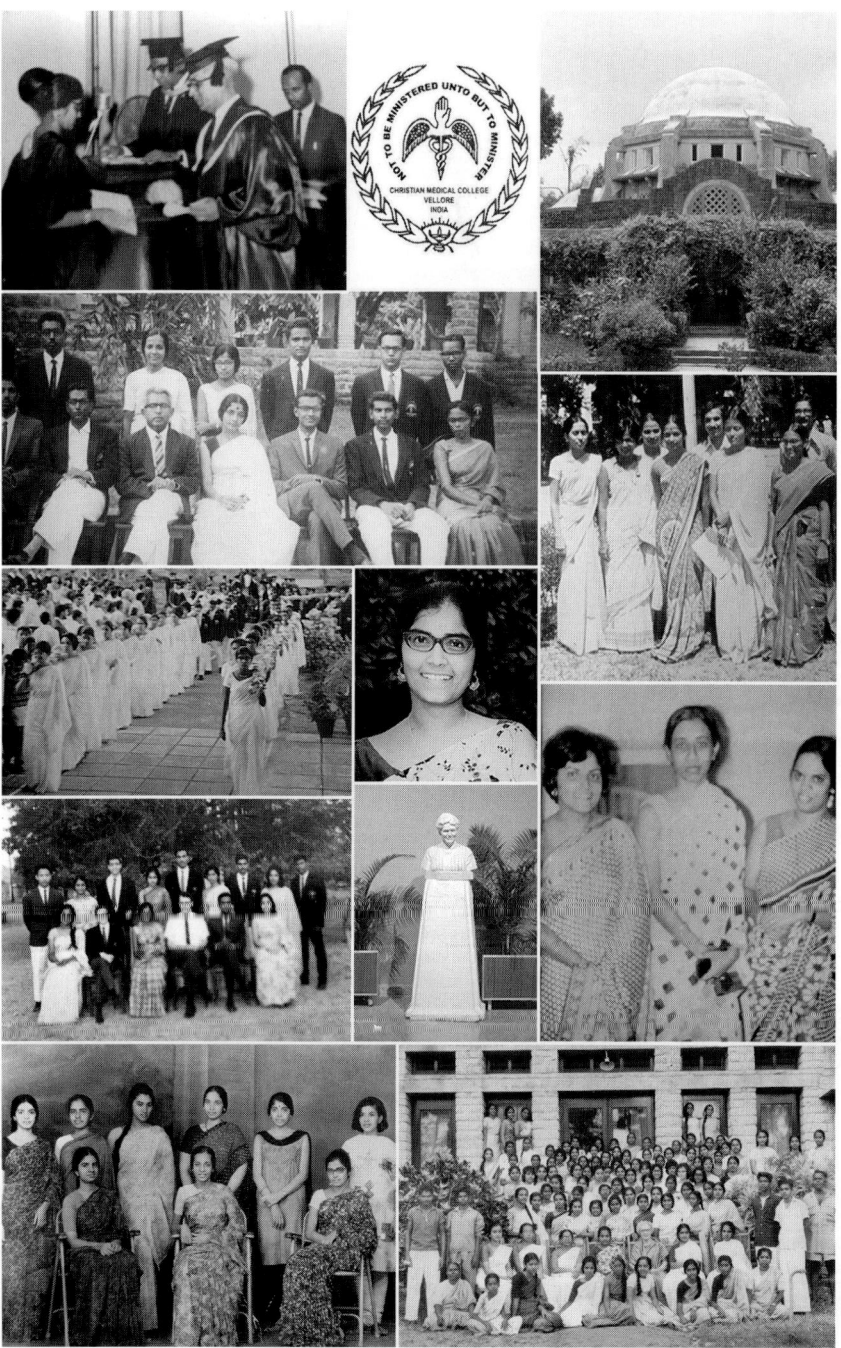

Christian Medical College, Vellore

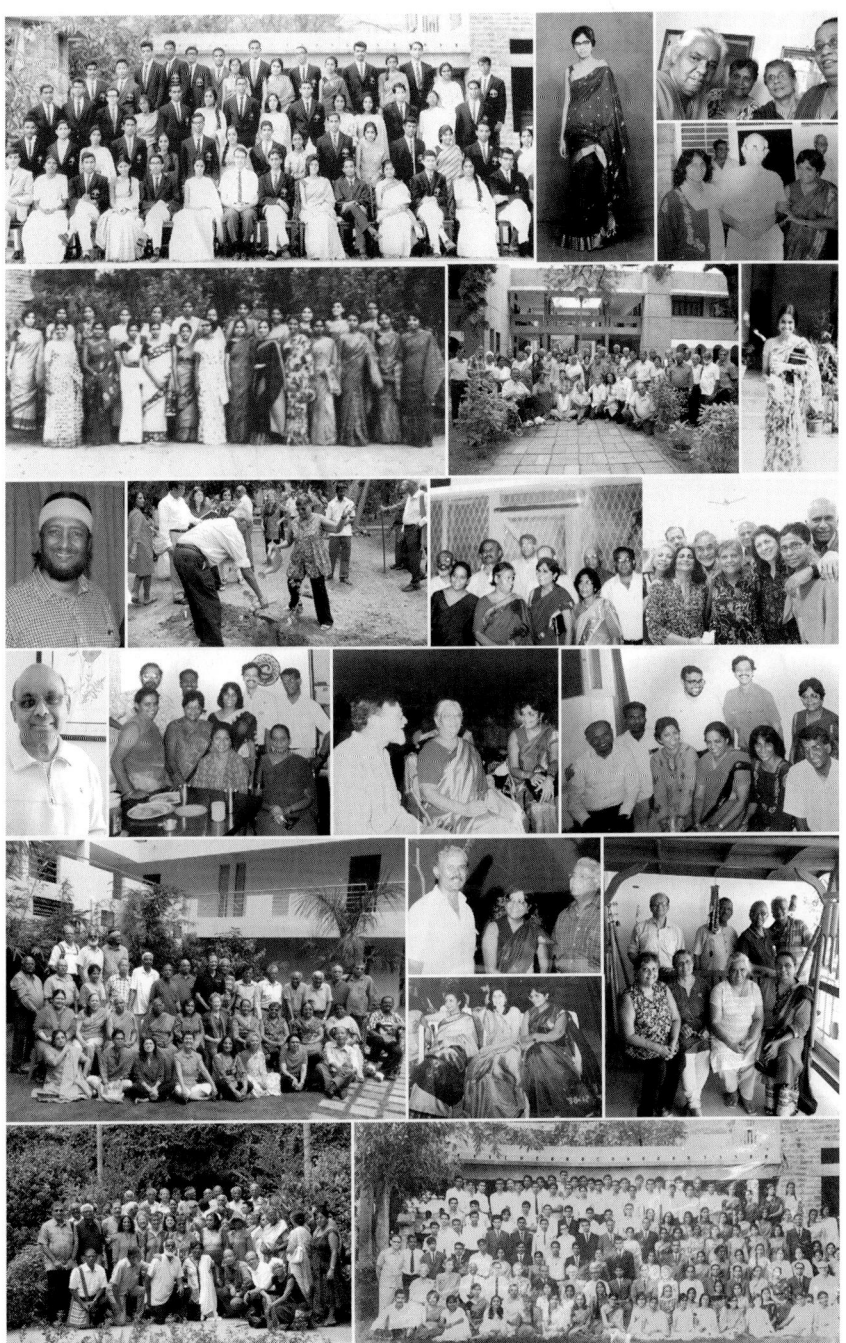

CMC Batch of 1964

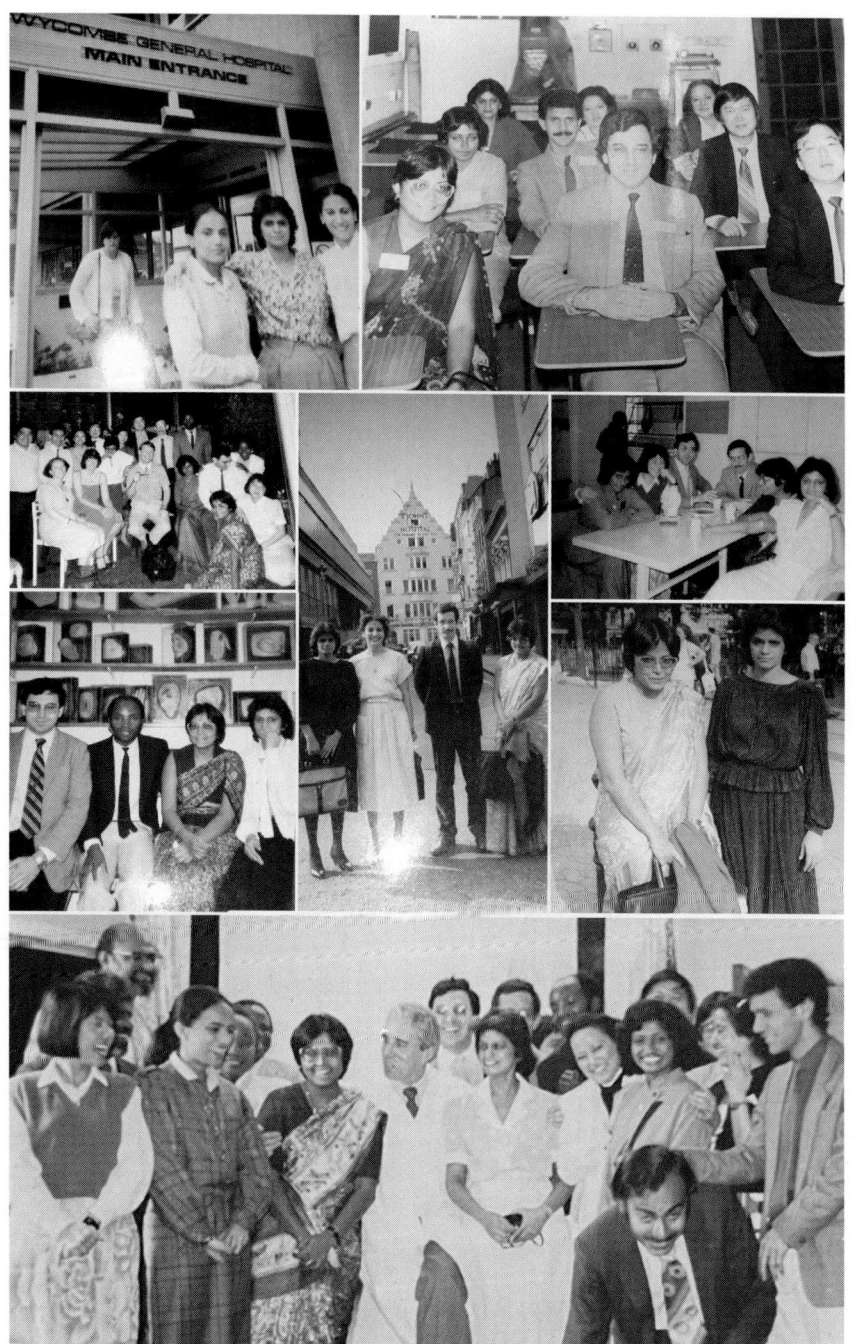

St Johns Hospital London

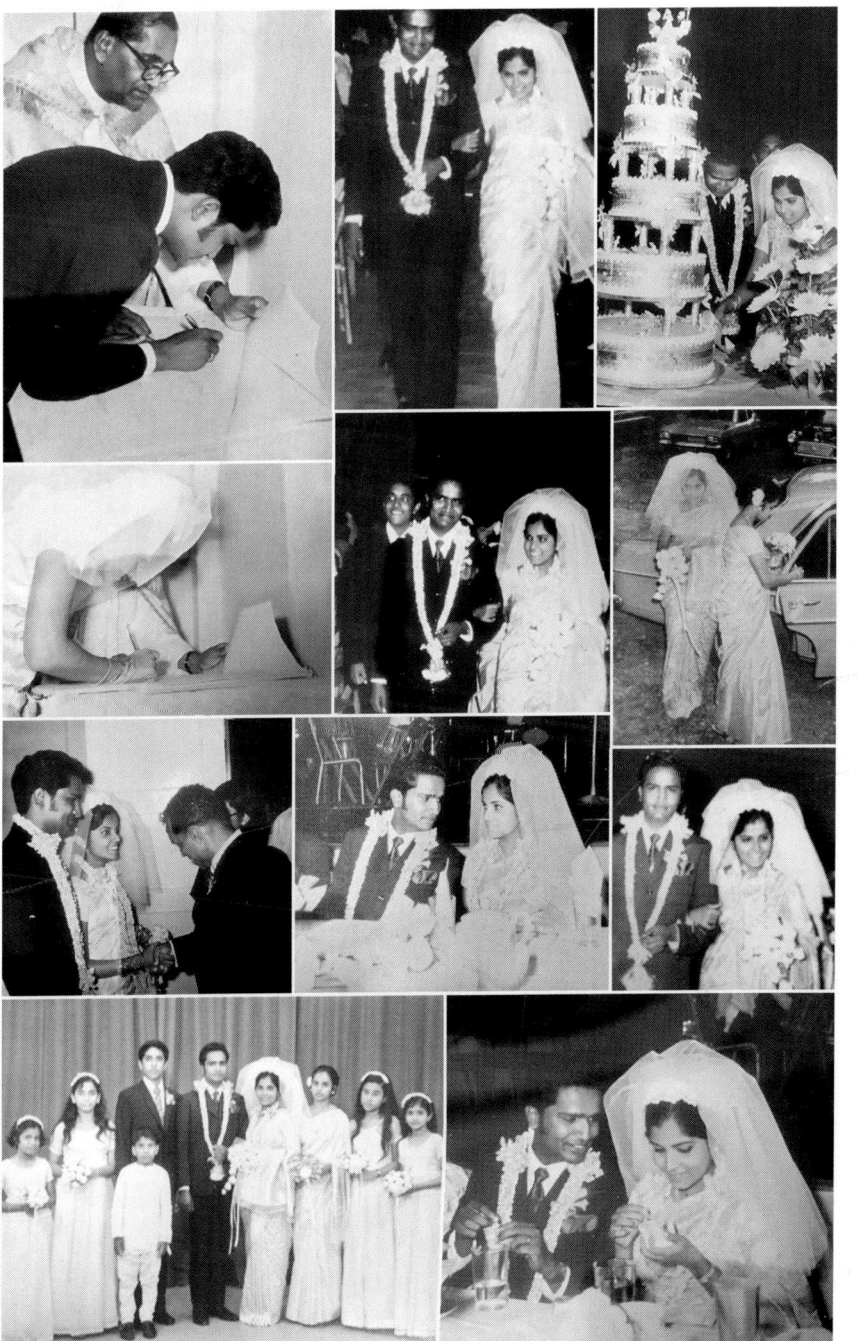

The Wedding

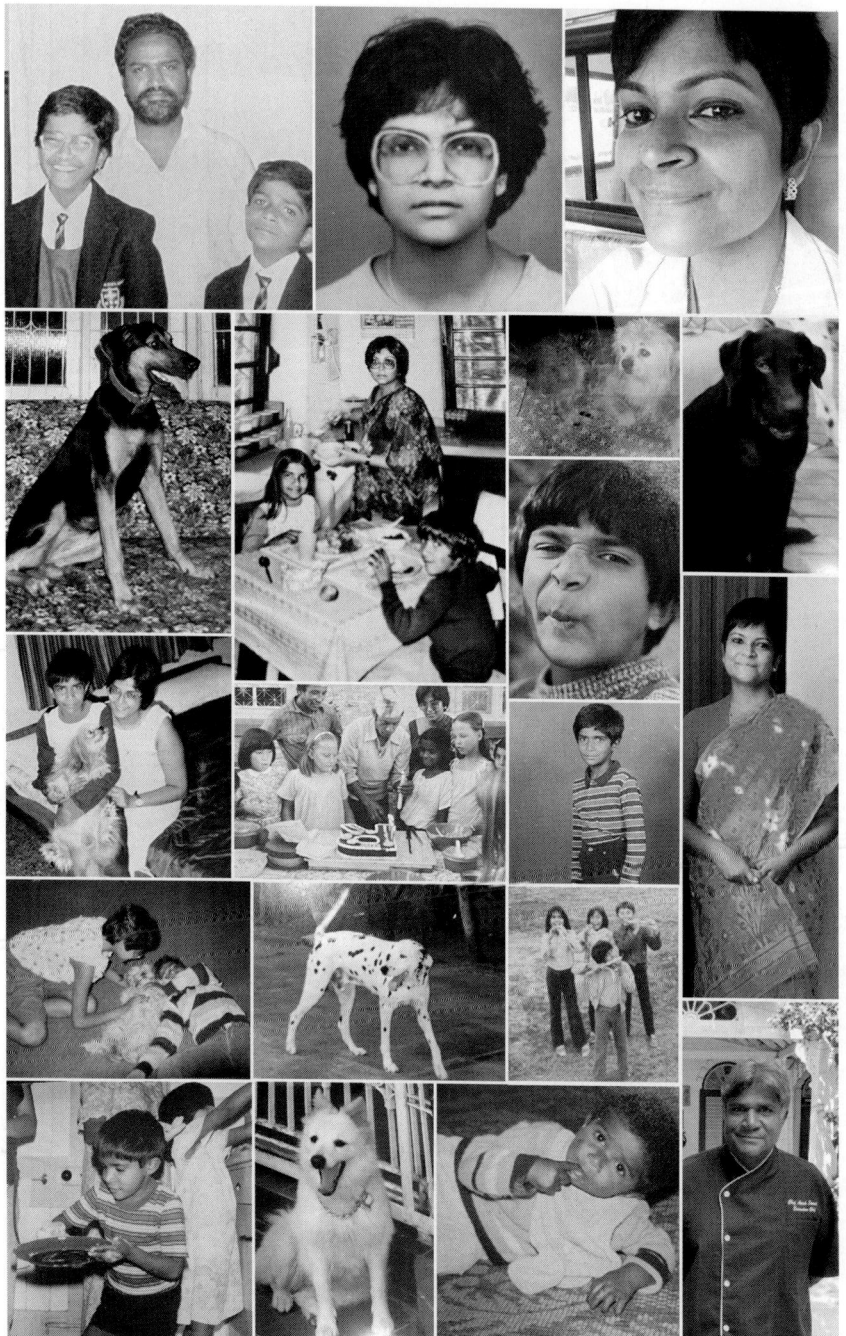

Kids 1

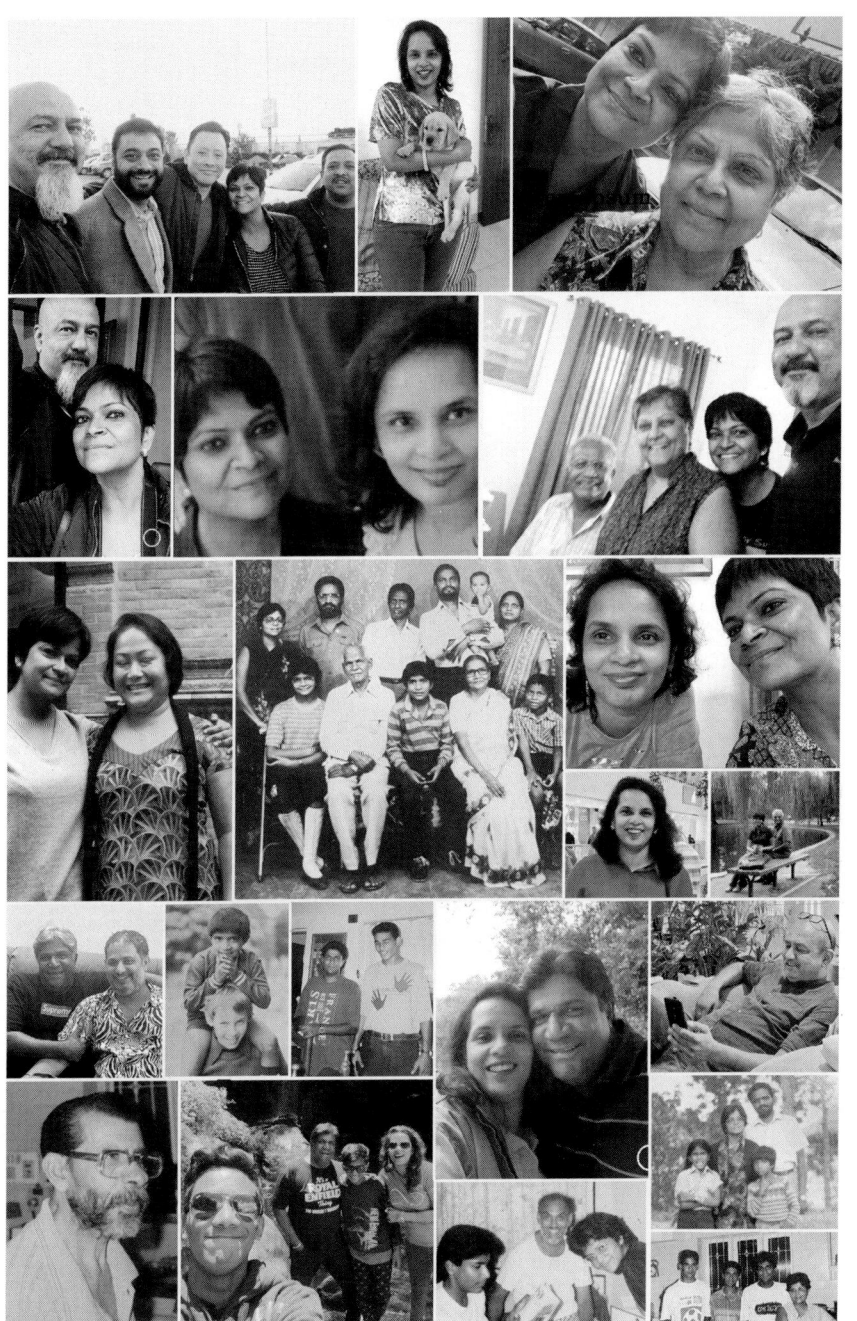
Kids 2

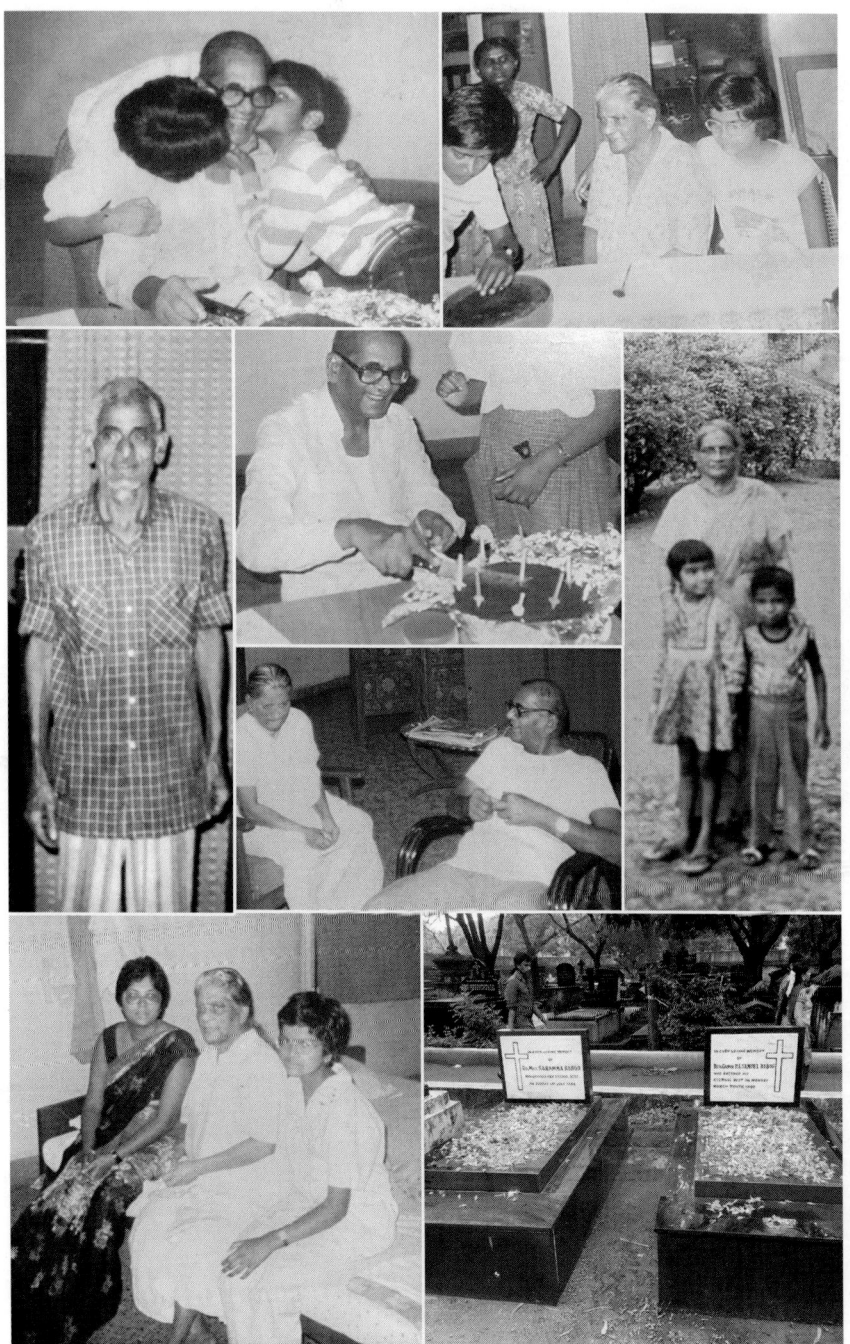

Retired and Relocated 1

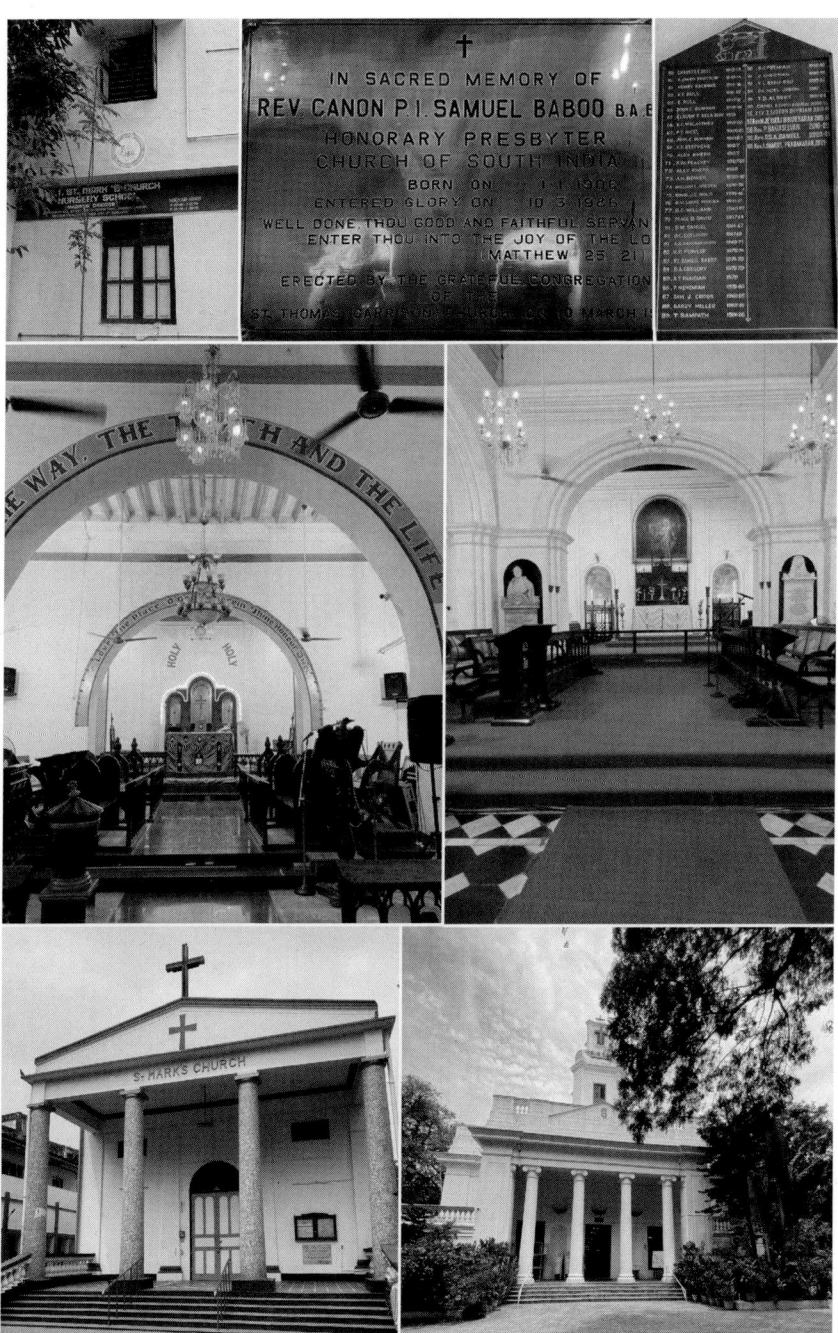

Retired and Relocated 2

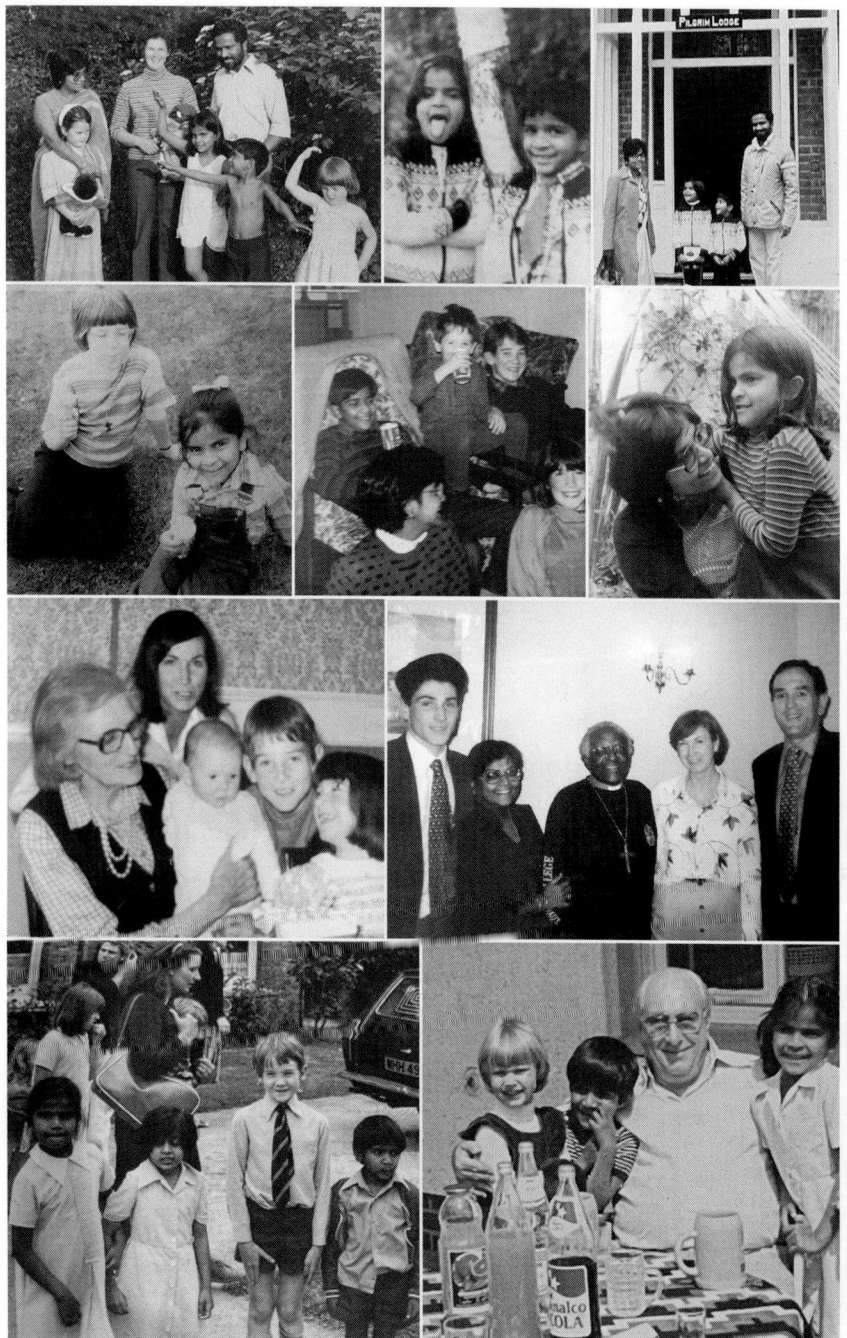

England

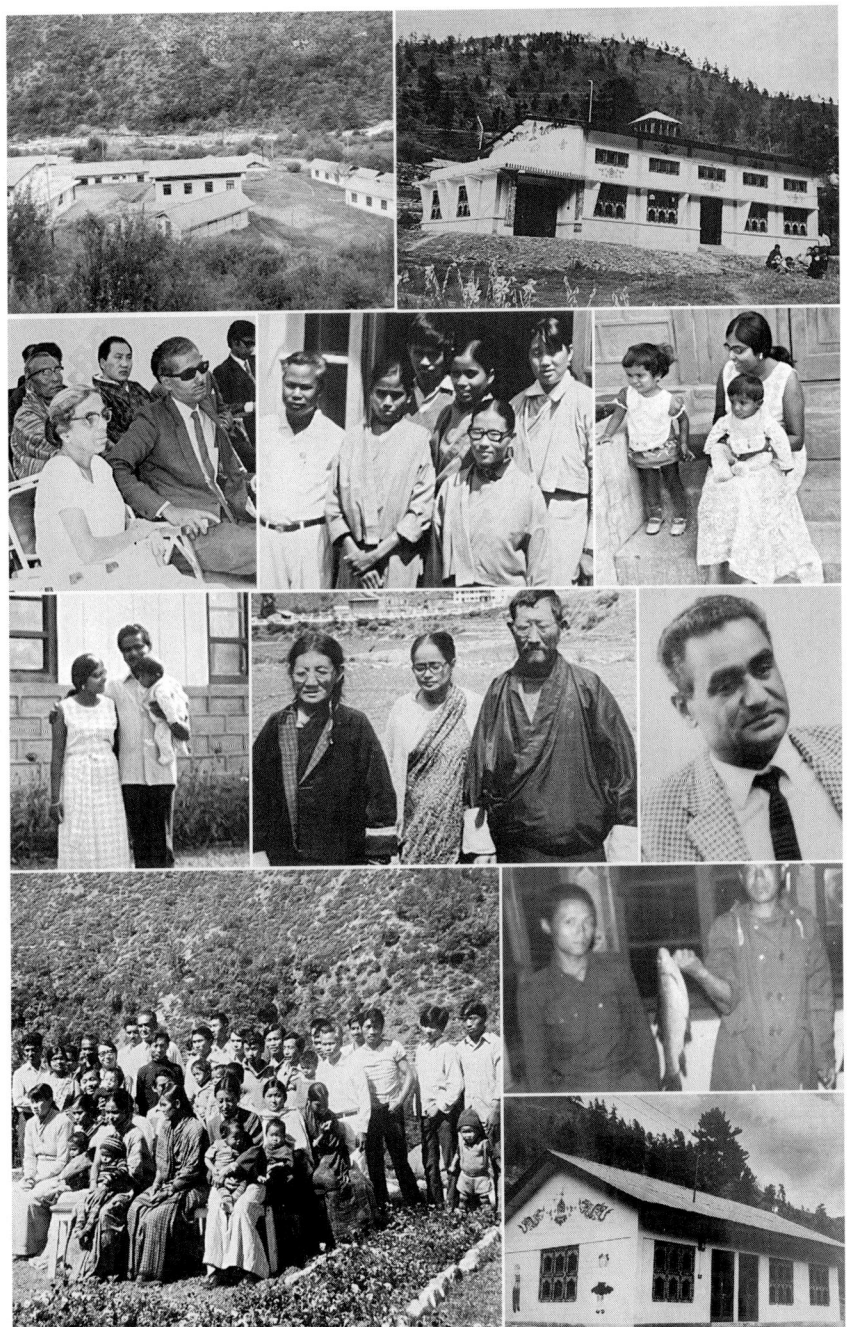
Gidakom Hospital Bhutan

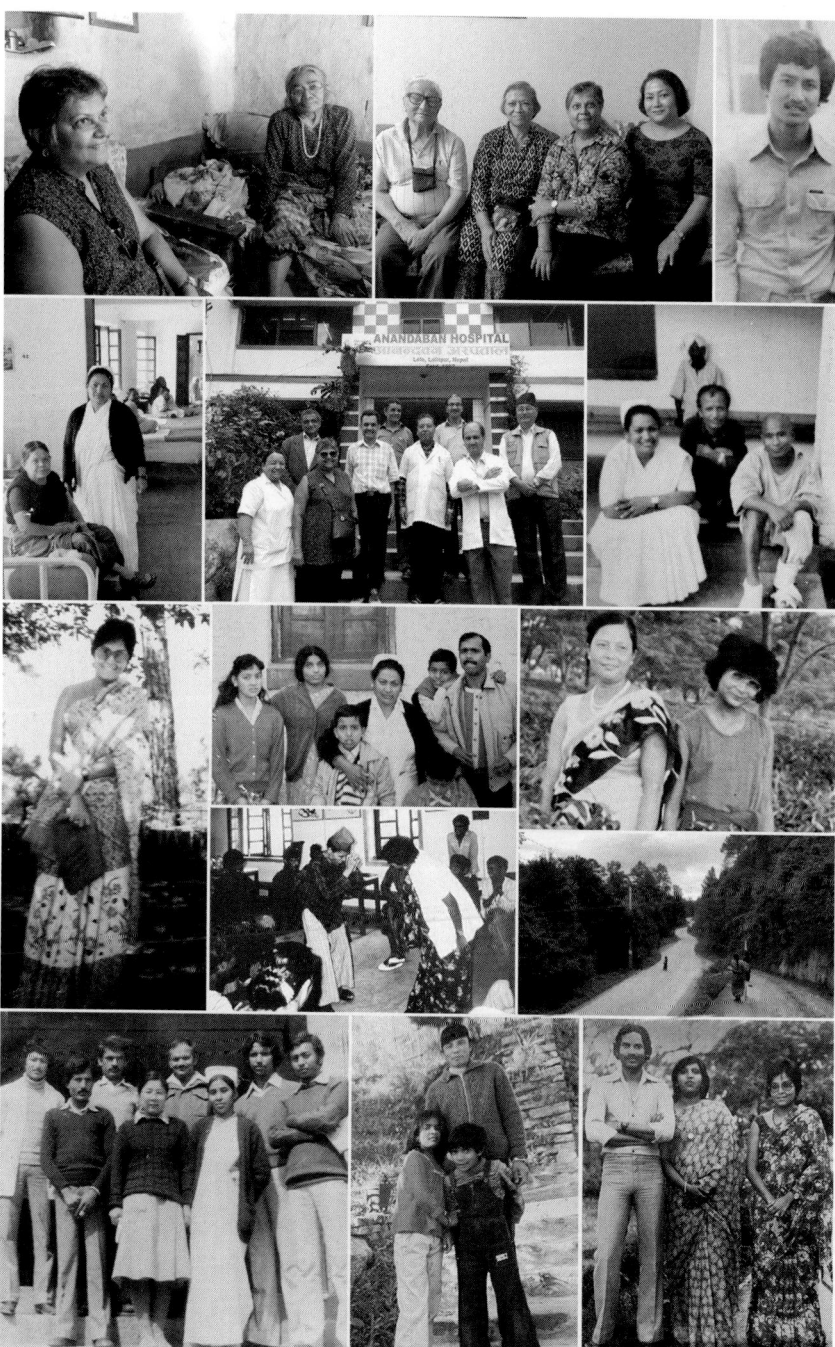

Anandaban Hospital, Nepal 1

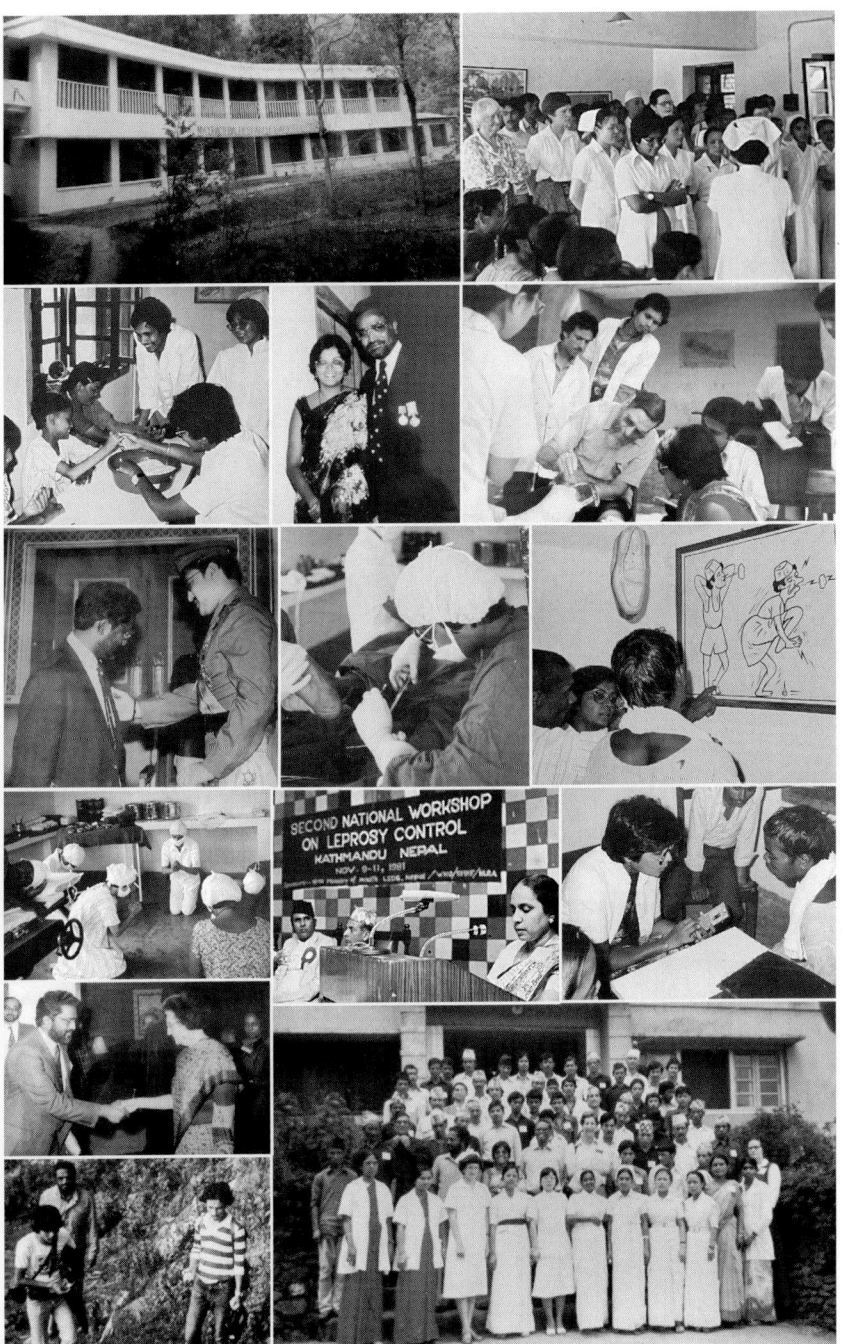

Anandaban Hospital 2

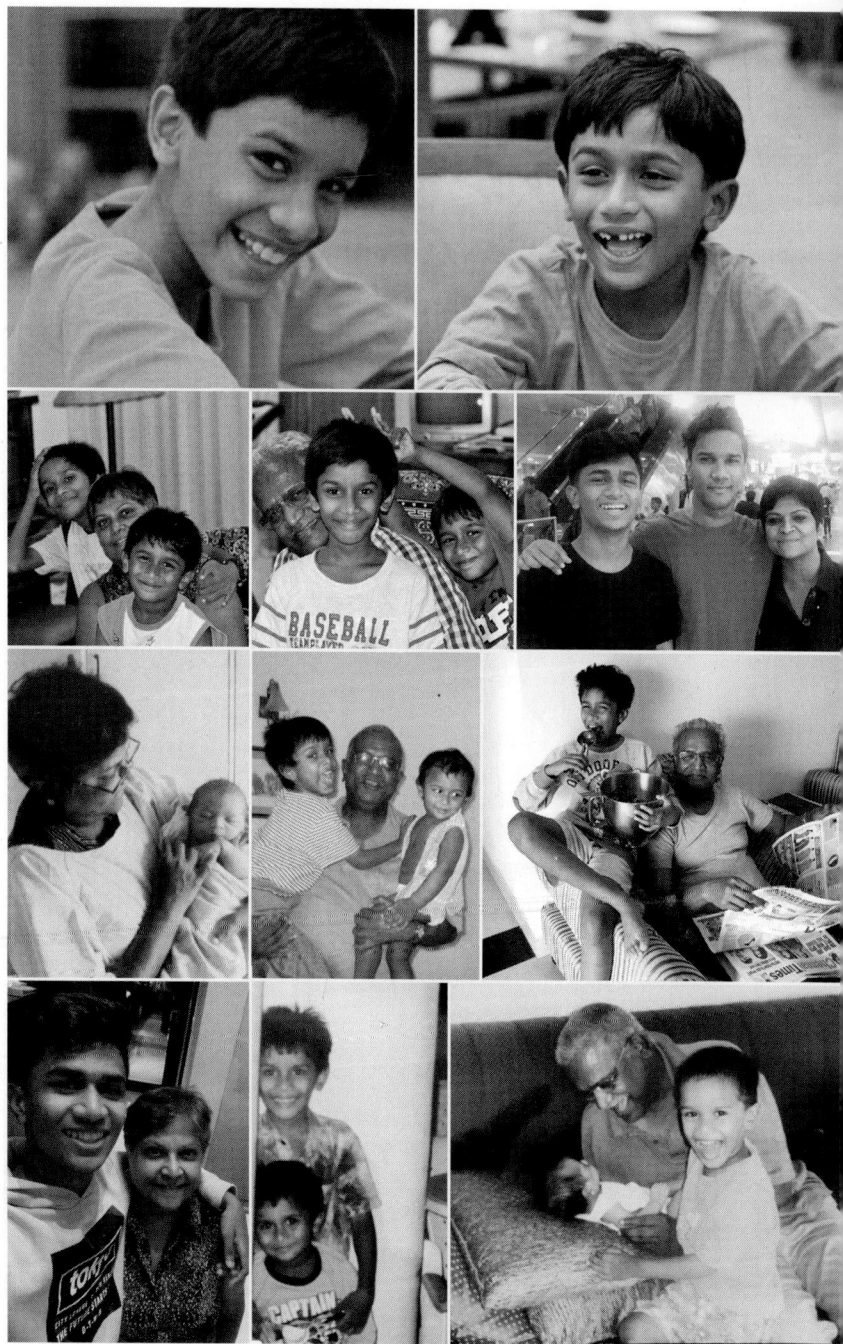

The Grandpeas Ashish & Rohan

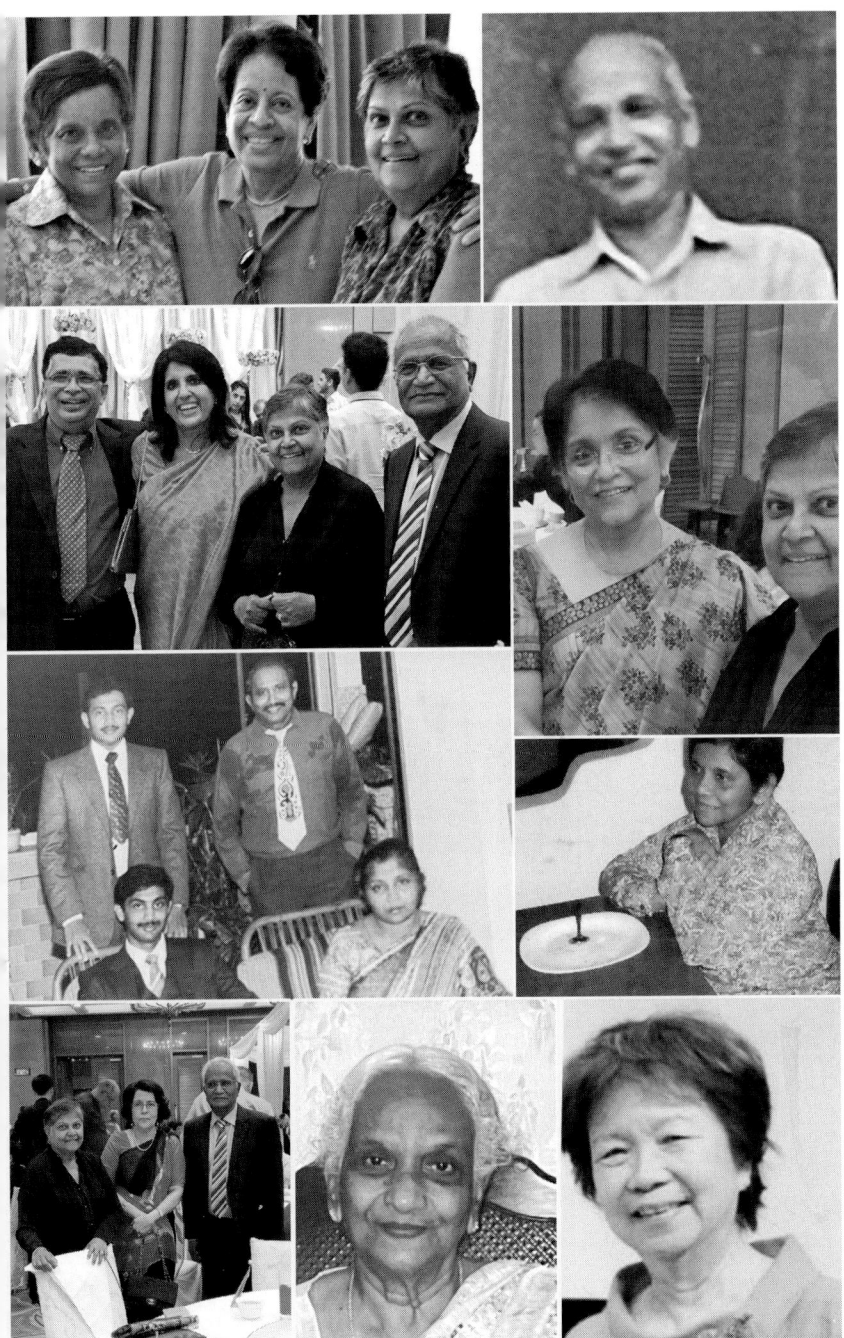

Singapore

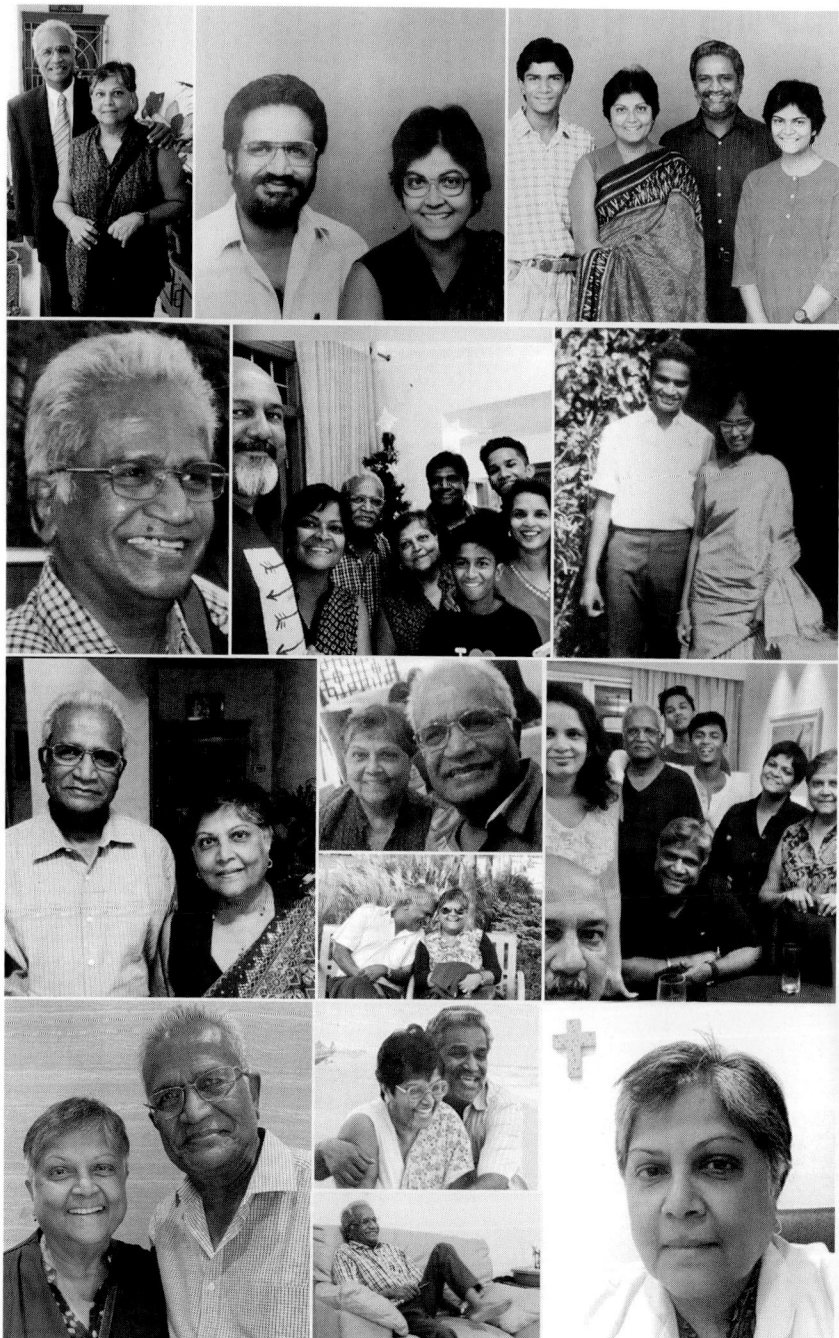

The journey

Epilogue
Thank You God